"... Dr. McGuckin sounds the alarm on deadly, costly infections and how to prevent them. Before you or a loved one heads to the hospital, reach for this guidebook. It could save a life."

—CECI CONNOLLY, former national health correspondent, *The Washington Post*

"Following on from her pioneering work in championing patient empowerment in healthcare, Maryanne McGuckin goes a step further in *The Patient Survival Guide* to give the patient the knowledge needed to make the healthcare experience a safe one. This book is written in simple language to demystify the 'coded' jargon for the layman consumer, but with all the experience of a confirmed and respected healthcare infection control expert."

—DIDIER PITTET, MD, MD, CBE, Director, Infection Control Program and WHO Collaborating Centre on Patient Safety; Lead, WHO Global Patient Safety Challenge "Clean Care is Safer Care"

"An informative book not only for patients and their families but also for the healthcare provider. This book should inspire us all to work together to prevent needless deaths from hospital-acquired infections ... (and medical errors)."

—Sorrel King, Josie King Foundation and author of *J   's Story*

"Receiving medical care at a hospital without acquainting yourself with the important information in *The Patient Survival Guide* is like jumping out of an airplane with no parachute and then hoping you grow wings on the way down."

—VICTORIA NAHUM, Co-founder and Executive Director, Safe Care Campaign

"The Patient Survival Guide empowers consumers to be active and effective advocates for themselves and/or loved ones navigating the complex healthcare system. A great resource for patient advocates and a valuable addition to every hospital waiting room!"

—BETH BOYNTON, RN, MS, Author, *Confident Voices: The Nurses' Guide to Improving Communication & Creating Positive Workplaces*

"This is the best book I've ever read that explains everything a lay person needs to know about hospital-acquired infections. If you want to survive your hospital stay without an infection, read it."

—ROSEMARY GIBSON, Author, *Wall of Silence and The Treatment Trap*

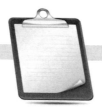

THE
PATIENT SURVIVAL GUIDE

*8 Simple Solutions to Prevent
Hospital- and Healthcare-Associated
Infections*

by
Dr. Maryanne McGuckin
with Toni L. Goldfarb

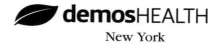

New York

Visit our website at www.demoshealth.com

ISBN: 978-1-936303-31-1
e-book ISBN: 9781617051180
Acquisitions Editor: Noreen Henson
Compositor: Diacritech

Medical information provided by Demos Health, in the absence of a visit with a healthcare professional, must be considered as an educational service only. This book is not designed to replace a physician's independent judgment about the appropriateness or risks of a procedure or therapy for a given patient. Our purpose is to provide you with information that will help you to make your own healthcare decisions.

The information and opinions provided here are believed to be accurate and sound, based on the best judgment available to the authors, editors, and publisher, but readers who fail to consult appropriate health authorities assume the risk of injuries. The publisher is not responsible for errors or omissions. The editors and publisher welcome any reader to report to the publisher any discrepancies or inaccuracies noticed.

CIP data is available from the Library of Congress.

Special discounts on bulk quantities of Demos Health books are available to corporations, professional associations, pharmaceutical companies, healthcare organizations, and other qualifying groups. For details, please contact:

Special Sales Department
Demos Medical Publishing, LLC
11 West 42nd Street, 15th Floor
New York, NY 10036
Phone: 800-532-8663 or 212-683-0072
Fax: 212-941-7842
E-mail: rsantana@demosmedpub.com

Printed in the United States of America by Bang Printing
12 13 14 15 / 5 4 3 2 1

In memory of my parents,
John and Anna McGuckin.

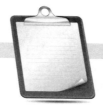

Contents

Contents

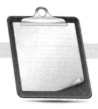

Foreword

Healthcare is an extremely complex industry and patients often end up seeing a different doctor for every part and organ of their bodies, from a podiatrist for their feet, to a neurologist for their brains. In the context of the hospital setting, this equates to many different physicians, nurses, and other healthcare professionals caring for one patient. Compound this by the many patients each professional sees, and you will realize how easily mistakes can occur and memories fail. The one person who can best manage their care in today's complex health care system is the patient. There is no mistaking that people will err, and errors can kill, yet teams can perform flawlessly.

Far too many patients are still harmed rather than helped from their interactions with the healthcare system. While reducing this harm has proven to be devilishly difficult, we have found that checklists help. Checklists help to reduce ambiguity about what to do, to prioritize what is most important, and to clarify the behaviors that are most helpful. Nonetheless, there has been some hope in recent years with reductions in bloodstream infections contracted from central lines used in the intensive care unit. While these lines are used to provide life-saving treatments, they require specific practices to prevent infection—a checklist and collaboration among clinicians helped to dramatically reduce bloodstream infections at The Johns Hopkins Hospital, in hospitals throughout Michigan, and across the United States. Clinicians have begun to develop, implement, and evaluate checklists for a variety of other diagnoses and procedures.

Yet, vigilance is unconsciously fickle; clinicians are distracted by competing priorities and unconsciously miss a vital step; too often patients suffer. Unfortunately, asking a physician or nurse to pay more attention is not the answer. There are no quick fixes and healthcare professionals need an extra set of eyes from patients—patients who are the central focus of care.

Patients can also use checklists to defend themselves against the major causes of preventable harm. Here are a few you can use:

Healthcare-Associated Infections

- Ask what the current rate of central line-associated bloodstream infections is in your hospital's intensive care unit. The best hospitals will have a rate of less than one infection per 1,000 catheter days (the definition provided by the Centers for Disease Control and Prevention). A rate above three should cause concern.
- Whenever clinicians enter your room, ask if they have washed their hands. Request that visitors also wash their hands often. Washing can be with alcohol gel or soap and water.
- If you have any type of catheter (tube), ask every day if it can be removed.

Identify Errors

- If you are admitted to the hospital, check your ID bracelet to make sure all of the information is correct. Every staff person should use this bracelet to confirm your name before any treatments or tests.
- If you are making an outpatient visit, staff should ask you to confirm your name and another unique identifier, such as your date of birth, before treatments or tests.
- Whenever blood or any other specimen is taken from your body, make sure it is labeled in front of you.

In this book, *The Patient Survival Guide*, Dr. Maryanne McGuckin provides an outstanding guide for patients. She details what patients can do to be part of the care team, to defend against errors, to help ensure they are helped rather than harmed by the healthcare system. Healthcare has a long way to go in reducing preventable patient harm; *The Patient Survival Guide* by Dr. Maryanne McGuckin points us in the right direction.

Peter J. Pronovost, MD, PhD, FCCM
Professor, Departments of Anesthesiology/
Critical Care Medicine and Surgery
The Johns Hopkins University School of Medicine
Professor, Department of Health Policy and Management
The Bloomberg School of Public Health
Professor, School of Nursing
Medical Director, Center for Innovation in Quality Patient Care
Director, Quality and Safety Research Group
Baltimore, Maryland

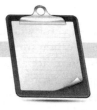

Preface

We all assume that going to the hospital will help us to recover from an illness or injury. However, going to any facility where a lot of other sick people are treated can result in patients *actually getting worse* before they get better, simply because they can catch someone else's infections.

These infections are called healthcare-associated infections because they are caused by specific bacteria or viruses that are present in the hospital and are transmitted to patients during their hospital stay. The infections are often spread by healthcare workers as they move from sick patient to sick patient, or by visitors who may have touched unclean surfaces in the hospital before going into a patient's room.

What most people don't know is that healthcare-associated infections are *preventable* if people who come in contact with hospital patients practice simple, well-known precautions. But if those precautions aren't followed and patients develop infections, the care they need is often difficult and costly.

I know this firsthand from my 35 years of experience as an expert in infection prevention. But when I began my career as a Medical Technologist at the University of Pennsylvania Healthcare System (UPHS), the field of infection control wasn't part of healthcare. Patients got infections, nurseries had outbreaks of *Staphylococcus* bacteria, and my job was to identify the bacteria so that doctors knew what antibiotic should be used. We would often see that other patients were getting the same infections, but there was never any questioning or thought that this might be a preventable problem.

Then in late 1970s major university centers such as UPHS established Infectious Disease Departments. When the UPHS department began a close collaboration with the microbiology department, I became very interested in this new field. I saw how my microbiology background would be valuable in helping infectious disease physicians track down infections and patterns of transmission. Thus began my career to identify and prevent healthcare-associated infections.

Armed with my advanced degrees, I entered the world of academia at the University of Pennsylvania, teaching and doing research with a focus on infections. I offered courses on preventing infections and conducted many groundbreaking studies showing how healthcare workers' unwashed hands might be the culprit in transmission of these infections.

In 1997, after 10 years of work on healthcare-associated infections, I realized that we were putting too much emphasis on simply identifying the problem. Each month we kept reporting how many infections we had found, thinking this would help to change the behavior of healthcare workers, in particular, physicians. As you will read in the book, it was then I knew that if we were to change behavior, we needed to involve patients, and we needed to begin with hand hygiene.

Why hand hygiene? We knew then, and unfortunately it continues to be true, that healthcare workers wash their hands less than 50 percent of the time that handwashing is required. We also knew that attention to these hand hygiene practices is the single most important way to prevent healthcare-associated infections.

During the next 10 years of my career, I conducted five major studies that were published in peer-reviewed medical journals, all sending the same message: "When patients ask their healthcare providers to wash or sanitize their hands before they have contact with them, hand hygiene increases and infections decrease." I called this effort "patient empowerment."

My message was quickly picked up by the media. (You can't tell people you are a superstar; you need to show them.) This brought a great deal of publicity for the University of Pennsylvania, and I was pleased that national organizations like the Centers for Disease Control and Prevention, the Joint Commission, and the World Health Organization gave recognition to my work on patient empowerment.

I believed that my findings would have an impact on the medical community, and to some degree, they did bring attention to the importance of hand hygiene. However, there was always a missing link: How do we get this information to the people who need it most—people like you, the consumer?

That's why I wrote this book. I want to empower *you* before you become a hospital patient. The power is in *your hands* to stop what has been often referred to as the silent epidemic—healthcare-associated infections.

I believe that the next significant change in healthcare will be driven not by laws, guidelines, standards, or programs, but by the demands of the consumer. I want you, the consumer, to know what I know about simple prevention steps you can take, so you don't wind up as "the infected patient." I want you to be "the empowered patient," someone who speaks up and demands proper hygiene during your treatment in a hospital or any other medical facility.

I assure you this is not a scary book about media-driven topics like killer super bugs and grisly descriptions of healthcare-associated infections that end with tragic deaths. Actually, it's mostly about people—consumers like you who generously shared their stories with me. Their lives were changed by healthcare-associated infections, but they all said one thing, "I wish I knew before I was a patient what I needed to do to prevent infections."

Many of these people expressed a sincere desire to inform others and help to make our healthcare system safer. In putting this book together, it was important for me to share their messages. My life has been enriched by their stories. I hope yours will be, too.

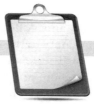

Acknowledgments

This book is the culmination of efforts of many colleagues, collaborators, and friends, who share the commitment to improve healthcare quality. It is through their time and enthusiasm that this patient survival guide was nurtured from concept to finished product.

I thank my colleague John Govednik, MS, for applying his technical and organizational skills to help the manuscript meet publication standards. It has been a tremendous help to have someone on my team who can turn publication technospeak into a set of in-house instructions for our team to digest.

I acknowledge the contributions of the following members of my advisory panel for consumer education: Eileen Cahill, Dorothy Daly, Joseph M. Govednik, Margaret Govednik, Joseph Karlesky, Margot Kleinschmidt, Michael Kutch, Thomas Malatesta, Lisa McGiffert, and Daniela Nunez. This team represents a wide range of professionals from the public and private sectors, which provided insight for chapter discussions and key points for readers. I was lucky that these collaborators provided me with *ten* different viewpoints to help perfect the message of the book.

I also thank my healthcare professional colleagues who reviewed the content of the material for completeness and accuracy: Jessica L. Bunson, MS, CIC; Lorri Goergen RN, BSN, CIC; Kathleen G. Julian, MD; Lynne V. Karanfil, RN, MA, CIC; Yves Longtin, MD, FRCP; Karen Ray, MT, CIC; Gwen Stewart RN, BSN, CIC; Julie Storr, BN, MBA; and Kathleen M. Vollman, MSN, RN, CCNS, FCCM, FAAN. They are the doctors, nurses, infection prevention and control experts, and colleagues from the World Health Organization, who bring patient safety to the forefront of healthcare quality training and education. They are the team who fortified this book with years of theory, practice, compassion, and empathy for the thousands of patients and their families who have been in their care.

Finally, I am most grateful for the contributions of my family. Thanks to my husband, John L. "Jack" Guinan, for his enduring and endearing support of my teaching, consulting, and now writing endeavors and our children (so called though quite adults now) John L. Guinan, Jr., Esquire, who so willingly advised me on contractual aspects of health writing and publishing, and Maryellen E. Guinan, Esquire, who contributed materials and manuscript writing for the chapter on law and healthcare for the book. It is truly rewarding that I, having always played the role of mother, professor, and referee, have now come to rely on their good counsel and perspectives for the benefit of my work in patient safety.

Of course, I would be remiss if I didn't acknowledge Buddy, our beloved Golden Retriever, who wears many hats around our house: entertainer, exercise reminder, and when accompanying me to the office, occasional foot warmer. With companionship like his through the seasons of writing this book, I can complete this project with my stress level normal and my heart warmed.

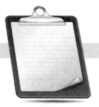

Introduction

Did you know that as many as 1 out of every 20 people develop an infection while they are in the hospital?[1] These are called "healthcare-associated" infections or "hospital-associated" infections. People didn't come into the hospital with these infections; they got infected during their hospital stay.

The U.S. Centers for Disease Control estimates that 1.7 million patients developed healthcare-associated infections in 2010 alone, resulting in almost 100,000 deaths per year. Patients with these infections need extra days of care in the hospital, which adds up to $35–45 billion in extra costs.[2]

Those are just cold, hard statistics. But when someone whom you know and love develops a healthcare-associated infection, it's a very different story. My friends and family know that I'm an infection control specialist, so I hear these stories all the time. Not just family, but often family members of patients would reach out to me at the University of Pennsylvania where I worked on research involving hand hygiene and healthcare-associated infections. That's why a woman named Teri called me in 2007, several years after her mother's death. She told me that an autopsy had been done, but she never received a report, and she still could not understand why her mother died. She was grief-stricken, worrying that she might have waited too long to take her mother to the hospital.

I told her how to get the autopsy report, and as I suspected, it showed that the cause of death was a fatal healthcare-associated infection, most likely sepsis (bacteria in the blood), which may have started at the site of her surgery. I can remember Teri's relieved call to me, saying how she finally could stop blaming herself for her mother's death.

To help you understand the drama and heartache of healthcare-associated infections, I asked Teri to tell the story in her own words:

TERI'S STORY: GUILT TO EMPOWERMENT

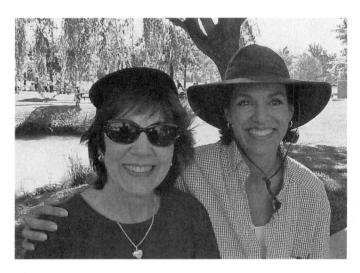

"I'll never forget Thanksgiving 2004, because it was the last Thanksgiving we shared with my mother, Barbara. She died the next day from a healthcare-associated infection. However, it took me three years of living with guilt until I would find out that was the cause of her death.

Two months before that Thanksgiving, she had been diagnosed as having bladder cancer, for which she underwent surgery six weeks before her death. The surgery was a complete success, so there was no need for either chemotherapy or radiation therapy afterwards.

Before her cancer surgery, my mother was the picture of health. She was a registered nurse who had worked at a blood bank for the last 14 years of her career. She walked daily for exercise, enjoyed gardening, and was a very active 70-year-old woman.

On Thanksgiving, six weeks after her surgery, my mother began complaining of nausea. She didn't have fever, diarrhea, or vomiting, so I thought she might have food poisoning. I called her surgeon, who didn't seem alarmed. He never suggested that I should take my mother to a hospital, but the next morning, I took her to the hospital myself. She died there 10 hours later from a massive infection.

This began my search to find out what went wrong. How had she acquired that infection? How could it have been prevented? It was only after I requested her autopsy report that I learned the results from her laboratory culture. It was a MRSA infection that took my mother's life, not the cancer for which she sought treatment. MRSA stands for methicillin-resistant Staph aureus, or what we now know as a "super bug," because of its resistance to antibiotic treatment.

Looking back at my mother's ordeal, I now realize many things that would have been helpful to know and steps that could have been taken to prevent the tragedy of her untimely death. Like most people, we assumed that reputable hospitals take every precaution necessary to ensure that their patients are cared for in a safe and sanitary way. After our mother's death, we found that this is not always the case.

In retrospect, I now understand what should have been done to reduce her risk of MRSA infection. She had an incision from her surgery that required dressing changes. Knowing what I know now about the dangers of healthcare-associated infections after surgery, particularly MRSA, I would have insisted that greater precautions be taken to ensure that proper sterile techniques were used during each step of her care. We would have insisted that each person entering my mother's hospital room would be required to wash or sanitize his or her hands and that all equipment in my mother's hospital room be adequately disinfected.

Had I been informed about the dangers of that type of infection, I was convinced that my mother would be alive today. Knowledge is power, and unfortunately, I wish that I had the knowledge then, so that I could have protected my mother from the thing she feared the most: a hospital error. I appreciate this opportunity to share her story."

SO MANY SICK PATIENTS, SO MANY GERMS

After reading Teri's story, you're probably wondering what causes all these serious infections. Sick people spread infection-causing bacteria and viruses into the air and onto anything, or anyone, they touch.[3] Hospitals are full of sick people, many with very serious illnesses, and all packed into a small area. This means that dangerous germs are everywhere. They hide on the surfaces of walls, trays, toilets, cups, instruments, and even ductwork. But the place they hide best is on people's hands.

Every time a doctor, nurse, medical technician, food server, or visitor touches an object, lots of germs go along for the ride. So, preventing healthcare-associated infections means preventing these germs from reaching other people. Hands down, the best prevention is handwashing and hand sanitizing. There's just one problem: Even though they know better, doctors, nurses, and other medical personnel frequently forget to wash their hands.

Three Ways to Reduce Your Risk

Being in the hospital is risky business. Nothing drives this point home more than knowing that thousands of hospital patients each year develop healthcare-associated infections. If you're hospitalized, you can reduce some of the risk just by knowing what to do[3]:

- Every time hospital staff members or visitors come into your room, ask them to wash their hands.
- Always wash your own hands after using the toilet or touching hospital food trays, medicine containers or cups, or medical equipment.
- When someone enters your hospital room, don't shake hands. Do you really know where that hand has been?

BUG WATCHING

As a professional in infection prevention, I've spent over 30 years of my professional life trying to get healthcare workers to wash their hands. You'd think it would be easy to just say, "Remember to wash your hands!" But research shows that's not enough. Busy healthcare workers are often so rushed that they forget to do what they know they should do. I've even seen this happen in the intensive care unit, where patients' lives hang in the balance.[4]

When I joined the teaching faculty at the University of Pennsylvania, I also served as a member of the hospital epidemiology team at the Hospital of the University of Pennsylvania. In 1979, I saw the need to train healthcare professionals in infection control. As a result, in my work at University of Pennsylvania, I developed the first national Master of Science/Doctoral (MS/PhD) program in infection control in the United States.

My training and experience prepared me for the challenge of finding better ways to prevent healthcare-associated infections. First, I focused on identifying the sources of these infections. Next, I had to find ways to eliminate anything and everything that contributed to their transmission.

I wanted to help Infection Preventionists know where to look, if they suspected that poor infection control practices were to blame so that the Infection Preventionists (IP) could take preventive measures before the infection could be transmitted to other patients. You will read throughout this book about the IP, the name used for the healthcare worker that leads the work of the teams to help prevent healthcare-associated infections.[5]

CHANNELING DR. SEMMELWEIS

I received many awards for these microbiology and infection control studies, including the American Society for Microbiology-Clay Adams Research Award. I was also the recipient of the Association for Professionals in Infection Control and Epidemiology's first national Bac Data Research Award, presented for the most innovative research in infection control. But, regardless of these accolades, those "bugs" kept spreading.

Then I remembered my medical history lessons. Back in the 1800s, doctors couldn't figure out why so many women were dying soon after childbirth. Dr. Ignaz Semmelweis, a Hungarian obstetrician practicing in Vienna, found the answer: dirty hands. Hard to believe, but in those days, doctors didn't wash their hands before treating patients. When Dr. Semmelweis insisted on handwashing, the death rate plummeted, simply because many fewer women developed infections.

With Semmelweis as my model, I dedicated myself to handwashing. Because I'm a research scientist, I designed studies to test several practical ways to increase handwashing, such as installing more sinks so they would be easily accessible to every healthcare worker.[6] I also tried posting bright-colored handwashing reminder signs in hospital care areas.

Despite all of these efforts, we found, as others have, that you can increase hand hygiene, but the effect is always short term. When the education efforts stop, staff members go back to old habits. These old habits continue. Today, we still find healthcare workers washing their hands less than 50 percent of the time.[7]

POWER TO THE PATIENT

Did I give up, or did I continue to follow my role model, Dr. Semmelweis? Even short-term improvement in hand hygiene might have satisfied some people, but not me! And it certainly provided no comfort to the many hospitalized patients who still were contracting infections.

What else could we do? Obviously, we needed more monitors, people who could always be there, who could serve as a constant reminder. Or as we like to say, 24/7. That was our "aha!" moment: We already had many more monitors: the patients themselves. What we needed to do was to teach patients how to be monitors. We wanted to empower them to become active partners in their care.

The solution: We told patients to remind healthcare workers to wash or sanitize their hands before touching you. And we told doctors, nurses, and other healthcare workers to heed those reminders and to thank patients who spoke up. When we tested this approach in our first four hospitals, we found that in just 6 weeks, we could increase hand-washing by at least 34 percent.[8] We then tested our idea at many other sites in the United States and abroad and found that our approach could increase handwashing by over 50 percent, and in some sites, up to 90 percent.[9,10]

That's why I wrote this book. I want you to know facts like this before you become a hospital patient. I also want to empower *you* to protect yourself by reminding nurses and doctors to wash or sanitize their hands before they reach your hospital bedside.

Your Reminder to "Bug" a Healthcare Worker

When you go to the hospital, take a little handwashing reminder that healthcare workers will see at your bedside. Here's what I designed to help patients "bug" their nurses and doctors.

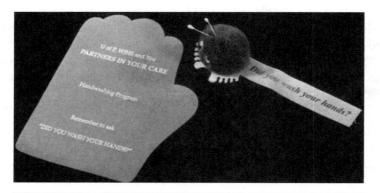

WHAT ARE THE RISKS?

Did you or a family member or a friend ever come down with an unexpected infection during a hospital stay? Unfortunately, many can answer "yes" to that question. People have numerous stories about relatives and friends who entered the hospital for simple procedures and wound up with serious infections that kept them hospitalized for weeks. According to the Centers for Disease Control and Prevention (CDC), more than 290,000 surgical site infections occur in U.S. hospitals each year. That's equivalent to 2 out of every 100 surgeries, which is 20 percent of all healthcare-associated infections The CDC also reported over 8,000 deaths in 2002 in patients with surgical site infections. An estimated 77 percent of these deaths were directly caused by the infection.[1,2] I don't want that to happen to you!

Infections occur even in the best hospitals. That's why all hospitals, big and small, are mandated by law to develop written procedures to prevent such infections and to take quick action whenever patients develop a healthcare-associated infection. They must also keep written records. What many people don't realize is that you can ask to see these infection records at all hospitals. In the pages ahead, I'll tell you how to obtain and compare infection reports from hospitals in your area to help you choose the safest hospital before you're admitted. That's empowerment in action.

But it's just a start. Once you enter the hospital as a patient, every procedure you have, everyone who treats or touches you, and every person who enters your room is a potential source of infection. If you've never been hospitalized before, you may be surprised at how many doctors, nurses, food delivery people, cleaning crews, and visitors come in and out of your room 24/7. It's hard to get sleep, but it's easy to feel vulnerable.

You can't let this information keep you from checking into a hospital. You have a greater risk of getting a serious infection while riding on a city bus or eating at a restaurant than you have sitting in a hospital bed. The difference is that you know simple ways to avoid infections in everyday situations. You wouldn't sit down on the bus next to a person who's continually sneezing and coughing. You wouldn't eat half-finished pizza crusts from plates left on a table next to you at a restaurant.

Of course, it's not quite that easy to avoid infections in complicated hospital situations like hip replacement surgery, childbirth, kidney dialysis, or the many other procedures that doctors and nurses perform. My job as an infection control educator is to make sure that these medical professionals are careful about preventing infections. The hospital staff members caring for you know what they should do, but they may be so busy that they don't take time to do it. You can help them.

Relax!

You have a greater risk of getting a serious infection while riding on a city bus or eating at a restaurant than you have sitting in a hospital bed.

YOU CAN DO IT!

Remember how guilty Teri felt 3 years after her mother died? There are so many scary books and reports about hospital deaths, medical errors, and massive infections that no antibiotics can cure. It's no wonder that people feel vulnerable and fearful of hospitals and healthcare providers. I don't want that to happen to you! I wrote this book to give you the knowledge and understanding to become an empowered patient and a partner in the fight to prevent healthcare-associated infections.

You need to think of yourself as a parent of a newborn. Remember how protective you were of your child, reminding people not to visit if they were sick, or how often you washed your hands and reminded others to do so? Why do I say that? It's because we have shown that hand hygiene compliance and the ability to empower patients are very successful in newborn nurseries and pediatrics units. Healthcare workers learn the habit of washing their hands more often, and parents, in turn, become empowered to monitor closely to make sure hand hygiene is occurring. You or someone who helps you as your advocate must take on this role.

You *can* do it! I know you can, because I've helped hundreds of hospitals in the United States and other countries to lower their infection rates by teaching patients a few simple steps about hand hygiene. You *can* take action to help yourself or to act as a spokesperson for someone else, so that you or a family member won't be added to the list of infection victims.

COMING ATTRACTIONS

Here's what this book will teach you. Each chapter explains common medical procedures that you may encounter in a hospital, such as surgical wound care, urinary and venous catheter use, tube feeding, and many others that present opportunities for infections to occur. The more you know, the more you'll know what to look for and what actions you can take to minimize your infection risks.

As you read, you'll probably have lots of questions. To make it easy, I've included FAQs in every chapter, along with simple answers that you don't have to be a doctor to understand.

I've also included four- or five-step prevention checklists at the ends of many chapters. These will jog your memory about simple actions you can take, such as reminding caregivers to wash their hands before they put on surgical gloves. Like airplane pilots, doctors and nurses also use checklists so they won't forget important steps in your care. As an empowered member of the professional care team, you deserve a checklist, too.

One more thing. Just as you take along clothes and personal items you may need in the hospital as well as your health insurance cards, now I want you to take along another kind of insurance card. It's a wallet-size card I developed to remind you about the 8 solutions to preventing healthcare-acquired infections that you'll read about in this book. You will find the card on the back inside cover of this book. Take the card to the hospital to quickly remind you about seven important things you need to do as a patient.

SHARING THE MESSAGE

From what you've read so far, you might think that this book is only about medicine and science. In fact, it's mostly about people. Over the past three decades, I've had the rewarding experience of talking to people like Teri and other patients and families who were victims of healthcare-associated infections. In putting this book together, it was important for me to share their messages. I also contacted several medical consumer groups and asked if their members were willing to include their infection reports. The response was overwhelming. The responders were grateful that medical professionals wanted to hear about their loss and apply those lessons to preventing similar tragedies in the future.

You'll read some of their stories in the following chapters. I also invite you to view my blog at http://www.drmcguckin.blogspot.com where you can share your own story and post infection prevention tips that may help other readers and their families.

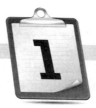

Enemy Invaders

Did you ever have a cut that took a long time to heal? The skin around the cut probably looked red and even felt a little warm. And when you picked part of the scab off—admit it, that's what everyone does—some yellowish pus oozed out. Yuck! An infection.

If you're a healthy person, your cuts usually heal without a problem. So, what went wrong this time? "Germs" got into the cut, and your body's defense system didn't fight them off fast enough. That's the simple, plain-English explanation. Scientifically, it's more complicated.

First, you need to know that trillions of microscopic bacteria (germs to you and microorganisms to scientists) live on your skin, in your mouth, in your gastrointestinal tract, and in other areas inside your body. Most of them cause no harm, and in fact actually help you maintain good health. Some of these bacteria hitch a ride into our bodies by living in the foods we eat. For example, some yogurts contain "live cultures" of bacteria called *Lactobacilli* that live in your gastrointestinal tract and aid digestion. Other harmless bacteria help you by just multiplying so much that they don't leave room for harmful microorganisms to survive.

A Word About Bacteria

Not all bacteria are harmful. Many are even helpful.

That's why some yogurts you eat are made with "live cultures" of *Lactobacilli*, which aid digestion.

1

Second, you're protected because your body's immune system works 24/7 to keep harmful bacteria, viruses, and other disease-causing invaders ("pathogens") from multiplying and causing problems.

Here are the basic facts about those germs living inside you:

Q: What exactly is a microorganism?[1]

A: A living thing that is so tiny that it can be seen only with a microscope. Bacteria and viruses are microorganisms. They are also called microbes.

Q: Are there other types of infection-causing microorganisms?[2]

A: Yes, fungi (plural of fungus), which are microscopic plants, and protozoa, which are microscopic single-celled organisms. If you bake bread, you probably use yeast—that's a fungus. If you've ever had athlete's foot, you can blame it on a fungus, tinea pedis. If you travel abroad, you probably know about the protozoa, *Plasmodium falciparum*, which causes malaria in people who are bitten by an *Anopheles* mosquito, the species that transmits the disease.

Q: What do bacteria look like?[2]

A: Bacteria consist of only one cell, but they exist in colonies containing numerous bacterial cells. They reproduce by growing and then dividing into two. Bacteria are in three shapes: balls ("cocci"; for example, Streptococci, the cause of strep throat), rods ("bacilli," such as *Escherichia coli*, a common cause of urinary infections), and spirals (for example, spirochetes, most notably *Borrelia burgdorferi*, which causes Lyme disease).

Q: What do viruses look like?[1,2]

A: Viruses are much smaller than bacteria. They're not even cells. They consist of molecules of DNA or RNA, which contain the virus' genetic code, all held together by a thin coating of protein. Most viruses are shaped like rods or spheres. They can't divide and reproduce. Instead, viruses act by getting inside the normal cells in the body and taking them over. Then the DNA or RNA of the virus causes the host cell to make copies of the virus. You've probably heard of the influenza virus, which causes flu, and the human immunodeficiency virus (HIV), which causes AIDS, and almost everyone is personally familiar with rhinoviruses, which cause the common cold.

Q: What's more dangerous, bacteria or viruses?[1]

A: Although both bacteria and viruses can be deadly, serious viral infections are more dangerous because they're more difficult to treat. Most—but not all—bacterial infections can be cured by readily available bacteria-killing drugs (antibiotics) that travel in the bloodstream to reach the infected areas. (In Chapter 3, you'll read about some bacteria that are especially deadly because they are resistant to antibiotics.) In contrast, viruses live inside cells, so it's hard for drugs to reach them. That's why it's been so difficult for scientists to develop effective antiviral medicines. Fortunately, vaccines are available to prevent some, but not all, viral diseases. For example, people with AIDS, caused by the HIV, must take many powerful drugs to control their disease. But as yet, medication has not been able to cure the disease, and no effective vaccines have been developed to prevent it.[1]

Q: Can antibiotics help people with AIDS and other virus infections?

A: Remember, viruses live inside your cells, where antibiotics can't get to them. So an illness caused by a virus absolutely should not be treated with antibiotics. However, many people with AIDS and other severe viral illnesses often develop concurrent (that is, developing at the same time) bacterial infections that antibiotics can help to control.[1]

Q: Then why do doctors sometimes prescribe antibiotics for people who just have a bad cough or cold?

A: Most doctors know that they shouldn't prescribe antibiotics for otherwise healthy people who have a new-onset ("acute") cold, bronchitis, or sinusitis (an "upper respiratory tract infection"). That's different from a long-term (chronic) infection. But even when doctors explain that antibiotics won't help some infections, patients often pressure them to prescribe antibiotics, and doctors give in to keep patients happy. Studies show that concurrent bacterial infections occur in only a very small proportion of people who develop acute upper respiratory tract viral infections. So skip the antibiotics when you have a cold, unless you have related medical problems.[3]

Antibiotics

Antibiotics don't work against viral infections.

A cold is a viral infection, so don't ask your doctor to prescribe an antibiotic when you have a cold.

YOUR IMMUNE DEFENSE TEAM

Getting back to your cut, the break in your skin allowed swarms of bacteria to enter an area of your body where they're not supposed to be. Some of those bacteria are the kind that are always present on your skin without doing any harm (they're called resident bacteria). Many other types of bacteria that don't live there permanently also land on your skin (they're called transient flora).When an opening in the skin gives bacteria—especially the transient ones—a pathway to get inside, there's trouble ahead.[4]

These invading bacteria attach themselves to healthy cells where they grow and multiply, causing damage to the surrounding cells. That's what an infection is: a condition in which harmful microorganisms start to multiply and interfere with the body's normal functioning.

If you have a healthy immune system that isn't weakened by illness or by side effects of drugs, it will immediately send out several kinds of infection-fighting white blood cells called leukocytes. These specialized leukocytes—neutrophils, monocytes,T and B cells, and natural killer cells—surround and destroy harmful bacteria and viruses. Sometimes this happens so fast that you never realize that you had an infection.[5] When you are in the hospital, your white blood cells sometimes don't work as strong fighters, so the bacteria aren't killed. These bacteria then will be able to multiply and cause an infection.

YOU'VE BEEN COLONIZED!

In earlier times when explorers arrived on distant shores, they often faced challenges such as harsh climate, illness, or famine. But explorers can be a hardy bunch, and soon their colonies started growing and expanding. Bacterial infections actually start in a similar way.

The first stage of infection is called colonization, during which bacteria find a way into the body (a "portal of entry") and attach themselves to cells (for example, the skin cells around your cut) or to tissues (such as the urinary tract, the digestive tract, or the respiratory tract). If the initial barrage of infection-fighting leukocytes doesn't kill the first bacterial "settlers," they continue to grow and multiply into increasingly larger colonies.[6] The time taken is called the incubation period.

Depending on the type of bacteria and the area that's colonized, it could take days, weeks, or even months before the spreading infection causes any symptoms. With your cut, you had classic symptoms of inflammation: redness, heat, swelling, and pain. Other types of infection could cause fever, nausea, muscle aches, sneezing, or coughing, to name just a few possible symptoms.

At the point when symptoms appear, you no longer have a simple infection; you now have an infectious disease that could possibly spread to other areas of your body. It's definitely time to see a doctor for an examination, perhaps some tests, and most likely, an antibiotic prescription.

It's Greek—or Latin—to Me![7]

Trying to wrap your tongue around the names of bacteria and viruses can be a challenge. Understanding the names is even more difficult. After all, most of them come from Greek and Latin words and from personal names of people who first identified the pathogens.

The following clues should help:

- Most names have two parts: a genus (the kind of pathogen) and a species (appearance) name. For example, *Escherichia coli* (better known as *E. coli*). The term *Escherichia* honors Theodor Escherich, who identified this bacterium. *Coli* comes from colon, the large intestine; *coli* means "of the colon."

- Some names are formed by combining two or more Latin or Greek words into one compound name. For example, *Rhodospirillum rubrum*. Rhodo is derived from the Greek word rhodun meaning rose; spirillum is from the Greek word spira meaning spiral; and rubrum is Latin word meaning red.

- Why are all the names of bacteria printed in italics, but not all virus names? Well…that's just the way it's always been done.[8]

WHY ME?

You eat nutritious foods. You do plenty of exercise. You sleep well. You are the picture of good health. So why did you suddenly get an infection from a simple cut? As Shakespeare might have answered, "Let me count the ways!" There are plenty![1,9]

■ First, you have to encounter a pathogen. The most common way that happens is through your skin, when someone touches you or you touch someone or something, and bacteria is passed on to you. Before you have a chance to wash off the bacteria, you may touch your mouth, nose, or eyes, which provides an entry point for the bacteria.

■ Maybe someone standing close to you coughs or sneezes and bacteria fly directly into your eyes, nose, or mouth, or onto your hands.

■ Do you have a new love interest? More than 500 kinds of bacteria live in people's mouths. Perhaps one of them got passed along while you were kissing. During sexual intercourse, you may have been exposed to the herpes simplex virus (herpes type 1 causes mouth sores and herpes type 2 causes genital sores). If you had unprotected sex, there's also a risk of transmission of gonorrhea bacteria or HIV.

Clean Your Hands!

Your mouth, nose, and eyes are good entry point for bacteria to get into your body. That's why you need to wash or sanitize your hands often.

If bacteria get on your hands—as often happens—and you don't wash them, guess where those bacteria end up when you put your fingers in your mouth, or touch your nose, or rub your eyes? They end up in your respiratory system, your circulatory system, and internal organs very quickly!

■ Perhaps you didn't keep your hamburger on the barbecue grill long enough to kill harmful bacteria. Several hours after eating, you started to feel nauseated.

■ Another possibility is you're visiting a friend in a city far from home or you're sightseeing in a foreign country. Although you've developed immunity to many pathogens common in your geographic area, you're now exposed to new pathogens to which you're more susceptible.

- Did you consider the season or the altitude? Some bacteria and viruses thrive in certain climates and locations. That could increase your risk of infection.
- Were you hiking in the woods? Check yourself for ticks. A tiny deer tick can transmit bacteria causing Lyme disease. Mosquitoes can also transmit pathogens.
- What about emotional factors? Are you under stress at work? Did a good friend die recently? Are you feeling depressed? Stress and emotional upsets can lower your immunity.

THE DOCTOR WILL SEE YOU NOW[9,10]

One more thing. Didn't you have a doctor's appointment last week for your yearly physical examination? Doctors' offices are loaded with bacteria, viruses, and other pathogens because so many sick people are there spreading their germs around. Not to mention germs on the doctor's examining table, the stethoscope, thermometer, blood pressure cuff, and other equipment, and on the doctor, too. The longer you stayed in the office waiting room—and possibly reading old magazines that have passed through many patients' hands—the greater was your risk of picking up an infection. Look at the doctor's hands below and on the next page and you'll see what I mean.

If a doctor's office presents so many infection risks, just imagine what might happen in a hospital. You'll find out in the next chapter, but first read Deborah Shaw's story about what actually did happen to her father when he developed a healthcare-associated infection.

Deborah Shaw's Story: The Last 3½ Days in the Life of My Father, Gene Shaw

I wish I had known what to do to save my father. He was admitted to the hospital on midday Wednesday, November 10, 2004, suffering from a severe blood infection (sepsis) that was due to leukemia. Less than 24 hours later, after being given intravenous antibiotics and a blood transfusion, he was walking around again, joking, and entertaining visitors.

However, by Friday, he was noticeably tired and coughing. Doctors were not alarmed by his cough. I was. By 7 p.m. that night my father was also alarmed, because he knew what it felt like to have pneumonia—he had a bout of it that spring.

Also, along with his bad cough, he had pain in his shoulder blade. That often occurs from a lung infection.

We had the nurse contact the on-call doctor repeatedly, but the doctor refused to come in to the hospital. By 2:30 a.m. Saturday morning, I had given up, after pleading, threatening, and cajoling the Nursing Supervisor. Nothing helped. We were watching my father die.

Finally, the regular doctors and nurses came in on Monday, but they could not work fast enough to reverse the damage that occurred over the weekend. My father, just barely 73 years old, was dead by 1 p.m. Tuesday, only 3½ days after our first plea for help, 2½ days of which we relied on weekend and night-shift personnel. Those doctors, nurses, and the hospital had completely failed us.

Some healthcare-associated infections are not preventable, even when the hospital staff and family members do everything possible. Mr. Shaw's leukemia weakened his fighting cells, so bacteria in his blood weren't killed and continued to multiply—that's what sepsis means. Sepsis is very difficult to treat. The death rate is very high, especially when the patient's disease-fighting cells aren't helping, as happened with Mr. Shaw. When the bacteria spread to his lungs, he developed the pneumonia that caused his death.

Was the hospital responsible for Mr. Shaw's infection? Did they do everything to prevent his death? You might argue that they did fail him by not responding over the weekend in a timely manner. But you can also argue that his immune system just could not provide support for him to survive, even if the staff had responded earlier.

So what could Deborah Shaw have done differently? In Chapter 5, you will learn what your rights are as a patient or as someone helping a patient (an advocate) and how to take matters such as this into your own hands. For example, you or your advocate can request what's known as a "rapid response call," which immediately summons a Medical Emergency Team of critical care doctors to the patient's bedside. Most patients don't know about this, but now you do. It is your right to request a rapid response, when necessary.

Although the outcome may not have been different for Mr. Shaw even if Deborah had known this technique, at least the guilt of not knowing how to get help or to be heard would not be part of her grieving process.

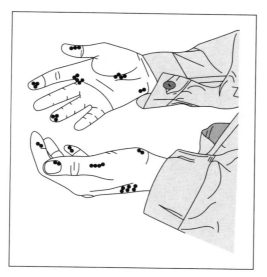

Doctor's hands showing germ areas (black dots).
(WHO Guidelines on Hand Hygiene in Healthcare.[10])

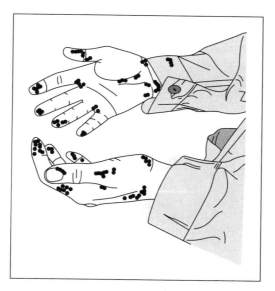

**Same doctor's hands showing how bacterial contamination
increases with time during patient contact.**
(WHO Guidelines on Hand Hygiene in Healthcare.[10])

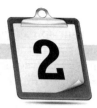

What You Need to Know About Healthcare-Associated Infections

Susan M. had a very painful left knee. Her doctor said that the problem was degenerative joint disease. He recommended a total knee replacement. No one likes to undergo surgery, but Susan was a healthy 64-year-old woman who didn't smoke, wasn't obese, and didn't have diabetes or other medical problems that could make surgery risky. She decided to have the operation.

As Susan expected, all of her preadmission laboratory tests at the local hospital were normal, and the fluid removed from her left knee showed no signs of infection. Her surgery was a success, with no complications. After 5 days of recovery in the hospital, Susan was transferred to a skilled nursing facility for physical therapy. She did so well that she was able to go home just 4 days later.

A happy ending? Unfortunately not. Several days later, Susan's left leg—the one with the new knee replacement—started to swell up. It soon got so painful that she went to the hospital's emergency room. At first, doctors thought she had developed a blood clot in her leg, so they started treatment with anticoagulant medications (blood thinners). That didn't help. But when they tested the fluid removed from her swollen left knee, they found that she had developed an extremely dangerous *Staphylococcus aureus* infection that wasn't controlled by ordinary antibiotics. (You'll learn more about methicillin-resistant *Staphylococcus aureus* [MRSA] infections in the next chapter.)

To prevent the infection from spreading even further, Susan needed surgery to remove her new knee joint. In the weeks that followed, she developed many severe complications that required repeated hospitalizations, blood transfusions, and continuing treatment with powerful antibiotics.

WHAT HAPPENED?

How could a healthy woman like Susan get so sick? Her surgery went well and so did her recovery. She was fine when she got home, so you might guess that she did something then that caused her severe infection. In fact, Susan didn't do anything wrong. Her hospital was to blame.

Like millions of other patients, Susan was exposed to infection-causing bacteria while she was in the hospital. It takes time for bacteria to become colonized in the body. During this incubation period, people often seem perfectly healthy. But if the body's infection-fighting cells can't kill the invading bacteria, the infection continues to spread. Soon the patient develops noticeable symptoms, such as pain and swelling. That's what happened to Susan. During or soon after her surgery, dangerous *Staphylococcus aureus* bacteria got into her surgical incision, became colonized, and weren't stopped by her immune system's infection-fighting cells. Susan had developed a healthcare-associated infection.

WHAT ARE HEALTHCARE-ASSOCIATED INFECTIONS?

Healthcare-associated infections are infections that people get after they first come into the hospital. In other words, they didn't come into the hospital with the infection or any signs of a developing infection. The infection was transmitted to them during treatment while they were there. Any infection a patient develops 48 hours after hospital admission is considered to be healthcare-associated. However, many healthcare-associated infections have a longer incubation period, so symptoms often take up to 30 days to appear.[1]

Acquired infections aren't caused only by bacteria; viral and fungal infections are common too. You can get any of these infections in many types of medical facilities, including intensive care units (ICUs), the emergency room, ambulatory outpatient care clinics, same-day surgical centers, and long-term care facilities such as nursing homes and rehabilitation centers.[2]

Healthcare-Associated Infections

Hospitals aren't the only place you can get healthcare-associated infections.

Infection-causing bacteria are also common in ICUs, the emergency room, ambulatory outpatient care clinics, same-day surgical centers, and long-term care facilities such as nursing homes and rehabilitation centers.

Q: Do many patients get these infections?

A: According to the U.S. Centers for Disease Control and Prevention, about 5–10 percent of people hospitalized in this country develop healthcare-associated infections. That adds up to an estimated 1.7 million people each year.[3] The studies show that about one-third or more of these infections are preventable, as Susan's was.[4]

Thanks to the new government accreditation regulations, hospitals are putting increasing effort into preventing infections. Nevertheless, a 2009 U.S. government survey showed that the total number of healthcare-associated infections has actually increased.[5] I believe that at least part of the increase may be due to the new regulations that require hospitals to report healthcare-associated infections, but the statistics do show that more work needs to be done to keep these numbers down.

Q: Are the infections serious?

A: Each year, more than 90,000–100,000 patients die due to these infections. As you'll read in the coming chapters, it can be very difficult to cure healthcare-associated infections, despite the use of powerful antibiotics. Even when people survive, they often need to spend many additional days in the hospital for treatment of the infection and related complications. The overall annual direct medical costs of healthcare-associated infections to U.S. hospitals ranges from $28.4–$33.8 billion, based on 2007 dollars.[6]

Q: How do patients get healthcare-associated infections?

A: Bacteria and viruses can enter your body through breaks in your skin and through mucous membranes in your mouth, nose, and vagina, for example. Medical devices such as urinary catheters and intravenous lines also can carry pathogens directly into the body. In the majority of cases, the infections are transmitted to patients by healthcare workers whose hands become contaminated with bacteria while they're caring for infected patients. The reason for transmission is that healthcare workers fail to wash their hands before and after contact with patients more than 50 percent of the time.

Patients in hospitals who fail to wash their own hands can also get infected if they touch dirty objects (a food tray, bedrail, toilet seat, or medical apparatus, or even a cell phone, for example) or from contact with people who have infections (such as sick roommates or sick visitors). In addition, infection-causing microbes can be transmitted through the air in droplets produced by sneezing or coughing.[7]

Wash Your Hands

Did you know that you can pick up a serious infection just by touching your hospital food tray or the railing around your hospital bed? The same goes for touching your sick roommate, or a visitor who has a cold, or even your own cell phone.

To keep safe and healthy, wash your hands and use hand sanitizer.

Q: Are certain patients more likely to get healthcare-associated infections?

A: Very young and very elderly people and patients who have had their immune system weakened by chemotherapy or an organ transplant are more susceptible. If you're very sick and are treated in an ICU, you have a more than 30 percent chance of developing a healthcare-associated infection because of your poor condition and the many procedures and tests you'll need. The more tests you need, the more chances you could come in contact with microbes on hospital equipment or healthcare workers.[4]

Q: So if I'm a healthy adult, does this mean I shouldn't worry that I might get one of these infections while I'm in the hospital?

A: Almost every person who is admitted to a hospital will undergo invasive procedures, that is, tests or surgery that can create an opening into the skin or an area of the body. For example, a tiny hole from an injection needle or a large open wound from surgery can let bacteria pass into the body. Tubes or catheters put into your body can also transmit infections. In addition, antibiotics you're given in the hospital to prevent or treat certain infections may increase your susceptibility to other infections. All told, anyone can get a healthcare-associated infection.

Fortunately, there are many ways you can protect yourself from these infections. The coming chapters will tell you how.

Q: Are there different types of healthcare-associated infections?

A: There are four major categories of infections:

1. Urinary tract infections
2. Respiratory tract infections
3. Surgical site infections
4. Bloodstream infections

Each category involves different types of illnesses, specialized medical procedures and devices, and particular ways in which infections can be transmitted. Urinary tract infections are the most common, followed by surgical site infections, but your personal risk of any type of healthcare-associated infection depends on the type of treatment or surgery you're having.

If you need to be hospitalized for a condition that could put you at a risk of one of these infections, keep this book handy and re-read the chapter about that particular category of treatment before you go to the hospital. I'll tell you what to watch out for and what you can do to protect yourself from infections.

HOW CAN YOU BE SURE IT'S A HEALTHCARE-ASSOCIATED INFECTION?

Almost everyone knows a relative or friend who developed an unexpected infection after being hospitalized. Sometimes anger over the pain, suffering, disability, and medical expense that results leads victims to sue the hospital and their doctors. As an infection control specialist, I occasionally serve as an expert witness in these court cases. That's how I came to review and file a report on Susan's knee surgery case.

I'll tell you more about infection lawsuits later in the book, but here's what you need to know now: Doctors often tell patients that everyone's body is home to numerous infection-causing bacteria and viruses, so there's no way to prove that an infection was actually transmitted by someone or something in the hospital. Don't believe anyone who says that—there are many ways we can tell an infection is healthcare-associated!

You Can Find Out What Caused Your Infection

Hospitals are required to find out what causes any infection a patient develops, and they know how to do it.

So don't believe anyone who says there's no way to prove that an infection was transmitted by someone or something in the hospital.

The truth is that hospitals are required to find out what causes any infection that occurs and to take action at all times to prevent and correct all sources of infection. They're also required to develop written procedures detailing what hospital personnel must do to watch for infections ("surveillance") and how to write full reports about infection cases. An official group known as the Joint Commission (formerly known as the Joint Commission on Accreditation of Healthcare Organizations) established these requirements and many other standards that U.S. hospitals must meet in order to retain their accreditation.[9]

Susan's case shows how these procedures should work, and what you should expect if you're hospitalized. To start with, before Susan was admitted to the hospital, doctors did blood and urine tests and checked her medical history to identify any illnesses, medications, or other factors, which could suggest that she already had an infection (such as an increased white blood cell count) or that she is very susceptible to infections (diabetes or use of steroid medication can do that). As you can see in the list on the next page, Susan had no presurgery conditions that suggested an infection problem.

Doctors call this a *zero* risk factor index. Does that provide absolute proof that any infection that Susan developed after she entered the hospital was definitely acquired in the hospital? Joint Commission standards say that hospitals must search for even more proof than that. For example, were there any problems during surgery that could have exposed her to infection? Susan's surgery wasn't unusually long (3 hours) and there were no complications, so that wasn't a factor.

The next question: Did Susan really have an infection, and when did it occur? As you'll see in the table on page 18, several tests and medical

Susan M.: Preoperative Infection Risk Factors

Condition	Yes	No
Recent hospitalization		X
Previous surgery		X
Steroid medications		X
Obesity		X
Diabetes		X
Malnutrition		X
Alcohol abuse		X
Remote infection		X
Skin disruption		X
Smoking		X
Elevated preoperative WBC		X
Abnormal preoperative urinalysis		X
High-risk ASA score		X

Abbreviations: WBC, white blood cell count; ASA, American Society of Anesthesiologists risk measure.

examinations showed that she didn't have an infection during the days she stayed in the hospital after surgery (postoperative stay), but evidence of infection was found within 30 days after her surgery (30 days is the standard of evidence in cases like Susan's).[3]

Case closed? Not yet. When I conducted my investigation, I examined the hospital's infection reports to check for anything else that might be important in Susan's case. I found that their surveillance procedures and policies failed to meet accepted standards. A Joint Commission on-site review of the hospital several months after Susan's discharge also identified several deficiencies in their surveillance and reports for various types of infections.

That's not all. In reviewing the records of patients hospitalized in the same room with Susan, I found that two of her roommates had infections that could have been the source of Susan's healthcare-associated *Staphylococcus aureus* infection. These bacteria don't travel in the air, so transmission most likely occurred when a healthcare worker touched one of the roommates and didn't wash or use a hand sanitizer before touching Susan.

Susan M.: Postoperative Indicators of Infection

	Yes	No
In the hospital		X
Fever		X
Elevated WBC		X
Elevated sedimentation rate*		X
Redness, heat, pus, and pain		
After discharge		X
Fever		X
Elevated WBC		X
Elevated sedimentation rate		X
Redness, heat, pus, and pain		

Abbreviation: WBC, white blood cell count.
*A blood test.

I concluded that Susan—a patient with an infection risk factor index of zero—developed a healthcare-associated surgical site infection that should have been prevented if the hospital had followed accepted standards for infection control surveillance and for timely identification and control of infections.

DO ASK. THEY'LL TELL

I've got fancy medical titles after my name—Dr. ScEd., MT (ASCP)—so do hospitals have to show me their infection records whenever I ask? Not so. In fact, with Susan's case, we needed a judge to order the hospital to turn over their records. However, you as the patient do have the right to see those records, without the need of any judge, thanks to the Joint Commission's accreditation requirements. It is public information, but you've got to ask to see it.

All accredited hospitals (and you really should avoid nonaccredited medical facilities) must have a plan in place to keep track of how many times patients get infections. The professionals who compile this information are called Infection Control Practitioners and more recently Infection Preventioinists (IP). As of March 2010, 27 state laws now require public reporting of hospital-associated infection rates; 12 of these states also have laws requiring preadmission testing ("screening") for MRSA infection and/or reporting the number of hospital-associated MRSA cases.

MRSA screening helps to identify infected patients even before they are admitted, so they can be treated with the appropriate precautions while in the hospital. This greatly reduces the risk that you could be exposed to someone else's infection. You can find current state-by-state updates on infection reporting and screening policies at http://hospitalinfection.org/legislation.shtml.[10]

If you don't have access to a computer, your local library can help you to check the information online. Or call your State Health Department, where a representative should be able to tell you what infection reports are available and can probably mail you a copy.

The table below, produced by the state of Colorado Department of Public Health and Environment, is an example of the information that is available to consumers. There is a table like this for each of the infection categories we've mentioned, showing whether the infection rates are acceptable, worse, or better than the national average.[11]

The table shows the number of bloodstream infections reported in hospital ICUs where patients are treated for serious heart problems that

Adult Medical Cardiac ICU CLABSI Rates

Health Facility	Location	CLABSI	CLABSI Rate	National Rate	National Comparison
\multicolumn{6}{l}{CLABSIs in the Adult Medical Cardiac Critical Care (Reporting Period: August 1, 2007–July 31, 2008)}					
Exempla Lutheran Med. Ctr.	Wheat Ridge	1	0.6	2.8	◑
Memorial Hospital Central	Colorado Springs	0	0	2.8	●
North Colorado Med. Ctr.	Greeley	0	0	2.8	●
University of Colorado Hospital	Aurora	4	3.5	2.8	◔

Note: The adult medical cardiac critical care location is an intensive care unit that specializes in care of patients with serious heart problems that do not require heart surgery. CLABSI stands for central line–associated bloodstream infection. Completely black circle, above national average; half black circle, at national average.

don't require heart surgery. Most of these patients need to have a tube ("catheter," which in this case is a different kind than a urinary catheter mentioned previously) inserted into a vein and then passed into the heart. These "central lines," called so because they go directly into the central part of your circulatory system, are a common source of bloodstream infections.

In this table, hospitals with a completely black circle in the National Comparison column are better than the national, average; hospitals with a half circle blackened are at the national average. A completely empty circle would mean the hospital is worse than national average.[11]

DOES YOUR DOCTOR HAVE THE ANSWERS?

If you're not a doctor or a medical expert, it's difficult to interpret infection reports. So, what can you do? It is very simple, you are now aware of these reports, so you simply need to make your doctor aware of the fact that you know this information is available and you want him/her to get the answers you need about infections in your hospital. If your doctor does not know or says don't worry, then you should call the hospital and ask to speak to some-one in Administration or to the Medical Director or Patient Safety Depart-ment or Infection Control Department to get the answers you need about infections at your hospital. For example, ask what they're doing to prevent healthcare-associated infections. Also ask how they did in their most recent Joint Commission (JC) infection surveillance report. Finally, ask how their results compared with those of other hospitals in your area and with the national averages for infection rates in U.S. hospitals. These JC reports can be obtained from the administrative office of the hospital.

If the infection rates at your local hospital are higher than for nearby hospitals, for example, it could simply be that your hospital is treating more patients who are very old or very sick. Or, it is simply that they are more stringent than other hospitals at gathering infection data. On the other hand, if the Joint Commission identified deficiencies that your hospital hasn't corrected, I recommend that you consider using another hospital.

Remember, hospital executives see their job as a business. They know their hospital is in competition with other hospitals, and they know that the public is already concerned about medical errors. As you might guess, if the hospital is in compliance with standards, hospital administrators will be more than willing to answer your questions. If they won't answer questions, take that as a warning.

Factors Considered in Choosing a Hospital

	Very important	Somewhat important	Not important	Don't know
Low infection rates	85%	8	4	2
Previous experience with hospital	54%	33	10	3
High staff-to-patient ratio	64%	28	5	3
Friendly staff	68%	27	4	*
Clean	94%	5	*	*
Close to home	49%	41	9	1
Good reputation	79%	18	2	1
Whether they accept your insurance	88%	7	3	1

*Less than one-half of one percent.

Several years ago, my colleagues and I conducted an Internet survey asking consumers to rank around 12 factors that they considered important when choosing a doctor or hospital.[12] We found that over 90 percent of people said it was important that the hospital looked clean. Over 70 percent said that if they knew their doctor or hospital had a higher than average infection rate, they would change doctors or not go to the hospital. You need to be in that 70 percent. In fact, I want to make that 100 percent.

Our research caught the attention of many hospital leaders because, as I said, they want your business. The table above from our Internet survey shows what consumers consider in making a choice about their hospital or doctor. How do you feel about these issues—are they important to you? Remember, going to a hospital just because it's close to you and easy for your family to visit, isn't really important. Better to choose a safer hospital and let your family visit you when you get home. In fact, having fewer visitors is a good way to help to prevent the transmission of bacteria and viruses.[12]

Q: If I need surgery, can I find out my doctor's infection rate for my surgical procedure?

A: You really do need to know what the infection rate is for your procedure and whether it is within what's considered an acceptable level. During your visit to the surgeon, simply ask what his or her infection rate is for that procedure.

Here's what to say: "For the last 100 surgeries like mine that you performed, how many people got a healthcare-associated infection? Is that higher or lower than the national average?" The answer should be in percent, like 1 percent, 2 percent, etc. If it is 1 percent, for example, that means 1 patient out of every 100 patients the surgeon treated developed an infection.

Make sure the doctor writes this percent information on the consent document you'll be asked to sign before having surgery. It could be important to know should you develop infection problems.

It is also important that you find out if the percentage your doctor told you is considered "acceptable." Your surgeon may not know this offhand, so you may think it will be hard to find out. Actually, it's easy if you have a computer or can ask someone to access this article for you from the Centers for Disease Control: http://www.cdc.gov/nhsn/. Once at web site check the section on Data and Statistics where you will find reports on hospitals and procedures and also be able to look at your State information.[13]

Print a copy of any report from the CDC and bring it with you to the surgeon. Ask the surgeon to look into the article to find the procedure you will be having and then show you what the acceptable infection rate is for that procedure. Now that you both have the facts, you can discuss this information with your surgeon. Remember, being informed means you are empowered to play an active role in your medical care.

Q: What if my doctor doesn't have information about infection rates in my hospital?

A: If your doctor or surgeon says infection is a rare occurrence or doesn't know the rate, I think you need to get a second opinion. Knowing about infection risks is an important part of the information that you need to sign in the informed consent form that is required before you undergo surgery. Receiving important information is exactly what informed means.

Q: I'm scheduled for elective surgery. Is there specific information I should ask about my hospital at the time I am going to be admitted?

A: Even when you've researched the hospital beforehand, be sure to ask your doctor if there are any current infection outbreaks in the section of the hospital where you'll be staying. If you're having major surgery, you may also need to spend time in the hospital's ICU, so it's important to ask if there are more than two patients in the ICU who have infections more importantly are there two patients with the *same* infection. If there are, ask to be placed in another unit, if possible, and ask what infection control steps are being taken in that unit.

Unless your doctor is an infectious disease specialist, he or she will probably not know all the answers to your questions about infections. Fortunately, hospitals are required to have one Infection Preventionist for every 200 beds. Ask the doctor to put you in touch with one of these professionals. Their primary job is to monitor infections and to prevent you from getting an infection. They will be able to give you all the information you need and will educate you on how to protect yourself during your hospital stay.

Healthcare-associated infections aren't inevitable. Some patients get them, but most patients don't. I want you to be in the "don't" category. To keep yourself safe, be sure to follow the rules listed here.

Rules to Follow

1. Remind all your healthcare workers to wash or sanitize their hands.
2. Remember to wash or sanitize your own hands when you are a patient and also remind your visitors.
3. Print the article that shows infection rates for each type of surgery and compare your hospital's infection rates with those of other hospitals in your area. Keep it in an easy-to-find place in case you need surgery.
4. Before you become a patient, learn about your state's rules for reporting and preventing infections. For example, some states require that hospitals do a culture test of every patientbefore admission to check for MRSA infections.
5. Familiarize yourself with any infection reports, Joint Commission reviews, and other information that are available to you from the hospital or online via your state's health agency. Consult your hospital's Infection Preventionist if the information in those reports is too complicated to understand.
6. Most important, please don't go to a hospital just because it is close to you and easy for your family. Check hospital records and choose the safest hospital within a reasonable travel distance.

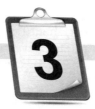

Attack of the Super Bugs!

Horror stories always get people's attention. Who could resist reading sensational news reports like "Invasion of the Super Bugs—Antibiotics Don't Help!" Pretty scary, right? Unfortunately, it's true. New strains of bacteria that ordinary antibiotics can't kill are spreading rapidly throughout the world, leaving critically ill and dying people in their wake. Like Superman, these "super bugs" often seem to be invulnerable. That's why medical researchers are urgently searching for the equivalent of Kryptonite to stop super bugs in their tracks.

What happened to create these super bugs? Where are they found? How can I avoid them? Keep reading for more on the latest developments.

WHAT'S A SUPER BUG?

Doctors have a wide assortment of antibiotic drugs that they can use to treat people who develop infections. But sometimes an antibiotic that has always worked for a certain type of bacterial infection suddenly stops working in patient after patient. That means the bacteria have changed ("mutated") in some way that makes them resistant to the antibiotic. This problem is known as antibiotic resistance. Usually—but not always—switching to another antibiotic will help to cure the infection.

Not all antibiotic-resistant bacteria are super bugs. Bacteria that rate this title are resistant not just to one or two antibiotics, but to almost every strong antibiotic currently available, including methicillin, oxacillin, penicillin, and amoxicillin.[1] That leaves doctors with only one or two super powerful antibiotics to try. Even when those antibiotics work, it can take weeks or months to produce any improvement, during which time super bugs often cause major complications or even death.

What's an Antibiotic?

Antibiotics are drugs that kill or limit the growth of infection-causing bacteria. Before antibiotics were developed, people very often died from infections. When penicillin, the first antibiotic, became available commercially in 1938, people called it a wonder drug because now infections could be cured. Since then, medical researchers have developed many other antibiotic drugs.

It's important to have a wide variety of antibiotics because some types of antibiotics are more effective against certain types of bacteria. Your doctor must determine what type of bacteria you have to prescribe an antibiotic that will be most effective.

Unlike *antiseptics* that kill germs on cups, glasses, doorknobs, and other surfaces (including your skin), *antibiotics* kill germs that live in your bloodstream. Antiseptics can be used frequently, but antibiotics are very powerful drugs that should be used only when absolutely necessary.

Antibiotics still save many lives, but overuse of antibiotics is costing some lives. That's mostly because antibiotics have been prescribed too frequently over time. For years, doctors prescribed penicillin for common ailments—sore throats, chest colds, and coughs—even though antibiotics don't work for these virus infections. Doctors know better now, but people who are sick enough to visit a doctor often demand "something" to help them feel better fast. If that something is an unneeded antibiotic, taking it may have the unfortunate result that bacteria in your body will develop resistance to the effects of that antibiotic. Then if you get an infection that really does require antibiotic treatment, you may find that the drug won't work for you anymore. I hope it won't be a super bug infection.

Antibiotics Don't Work for a Cold

Did you know that antibiotics don't work to cure the common cold? That's because colds are caused by viruses not by bacteria. Antibiotics don't kill viruses. Doctors know this, but sometimes they give in when sneezing patients demand a prescription for antibiotics because "maybe there's a chance it will help." Please don't take that foolish chance!

MEET THE SUPER BUGS

The following are the three most common super bugs:

- Methicillin-resistant *Staphylococcus aureus* (MRSA)
- Vancomycin-resistant *Enterococcus* (VRE)
- *Clostridium difficile* ("*C. diff*")

MRSA was the first super bug infection to make news headlines. Back in the 1970s, doctors were alarmed to encounter patients dying from seemingly ordinary "*Staph*" infections that couldn't be controlled with any of the penicillin-like antibiotics known as beta-lactams, including penicillin, amoxicillin, oxacillin, methicillin, and others.[2]

MRSA is an especially dangerous category of *Staph*, not just because of antibiotic resistance but because MRSA can spread rapidly throughout the body, causing life-threatening harm to numerous organs.[3] Antibiotics such as vancomycin and rifampin often work to control MRSA in hospitalized patients.[4] When other antibiotics fail to work, newer antibiotics such as linezolid, daptomycin, and tigecycline are now being used for MRSA.[5]

Almost everyone has *S. aureus* on their skin and in their nostrils. Although it usually isn't harmful, *Staph* can cause common skin infections such as boils and abscesses that are easy to treat.[6] But especially in hospitalized patients who have had surgery or medical procedures, *Staph* can lead to potentially fatal antibiotic-resistant infections in surgical incisions, heart valves, and places where tubes have been inserted into the body.

Serious antibiotic-resistant *Staph* infections are also on the increase in healthy, nonhospitalized people—especially children and sometimes with fatal results.[7] Young athletes such as football players and wrestlers can also contract MRSA from close skin-to-skin contact with other athletes who don't realize that pimples or boils on their skin are infected with *Staph*.[8]

VRE, the second super bug, was initially detected in the late 1980s. Because many types of *Staph* bacteria had become resistant to methicillin, doctors increased their use of a different type of antibiotic, vancomycin. Unfortunately, bacterial resistance to vancomycin soon developed, this time in enterococci bacteria such as *Enterococcus faecium* and *Enterococcus faecalis*, which are commonly found in the gastrointestinal tract and, in women, the genital tract.[9] Soon some *Staph* bacteria also developed vancomycin resistance.

Enterococci usually cause little problem in healthy people. But as with MRSA, hospitalized patients are more susceptible to the VRE super bug. Despite the risk of resistance, intravenously administered vancomycin is still the most useful antibiotic for many of these infections. However, even when the drug works initially, enterococci bacteria may develop vancomycin resistance during treatment.[10]

C. diff is another common type of bacteria that we all have in our intestinal tract. *C. diff* usually lives peacefully along with many good intestinal bacteria that stimulate the immune system and help to control harmful bacteria. When you take an antibiotic to kill bacteria that are causing an infection, sometimes these good bacteria are killed along with the bad ones. Without good bacteria to control it, *C. diff* quickly multiplies, releasing harmful substances called toxins.[11] This leads to production of cells that eat away the lining of the colon, causing severe diarrhea and colitis (inflammation of the colon).[12]

People infected with *C. diff* excrete spores containing the bacteria in their feces. Hand sanitizers don't kill these spores, so frequent handwashing is the best protection against spread of *C. diff*. It's also important to thoroughly clean all surfaces in an infected patient's room, because any surface that comes in contact with even a tiny spot of fecal matter can provide a way for *C. diff* spores to be transferred to people who touch that surface.[13] Another way to prevent contact with fecal spores is using disposable rectal thermometers for infected patients, rather than the electronic thermometers that are reused for many patients.[14]

Studies show that 90 percent of *C. diff* infections occur in people who recently took antibiotics for non-*C. diff* infections. Elderly hospitalized patients are the most frequent victims.[15] For people who develop *C. diff* infections while they're taking antibiotics for a non-*C. diff* infection, stopping antibiotic treatment frequently helps to cure the *C. diff* infection.

Many *C. diff* infections can be treated with the antibiotics such as metronidazole or vancomycin, but *C. diff* resistance is rapidly increasing.[16] This qualifies *C. diff* for super bug status.

Q: Why do we call these bacteria super bugs?

A: They're called super bugs primarily because the media gave them that name. But their super strength in resisting strong antibiotics definitely merits the super bug title.

Q: There are lots of different antibiotics. Why can't doctors find some that work against super bugs?

A: Although their names might suggest that they are resistant to only one antibiotic—for example, methicillin-resistant (MRSA) and vancomycin-resistant (VRE)—these super bugs are resistant to most antibiotics. At first, doctors feared that they had run out of antibiotics to try. Today, thanks to recently developed drugs, we do have some added antibiotic options. Because of this, super bugs are now commonly referred to as "multidrug-resistant pathogens" (MDRPs).

Q: Does that mean super bug infections are curable now?

A: Infections caused by multidrug-resistant bacteria produce the same kind of symptoms as do easily treatable infections with other bacteria. The difference is that doctors have markedly fewer antibiotic choices for fighting these super bugs. Even when one of the newer antibiotics seems to work, the super bug may soon develop resistance to it, giving time to the infection to spread and cause damage. There are many successful cures, but also many uncontrollable super bug infections that end in death.

Q: Why do super bugs become resistant to antibiotics?

A: Bacteria can change in several ways that reduce or totally eliminate their susceptibility to antibiotics. One way is a genetic "accident" (a mutation), similar to what causes some babies to be born with an abnormal heart or even six fingers on each hand. For bacteria, gene mutations can make the mutant bacteria unusually resistant to antibiotics.

Another cause of bacterial resistance is more common than mutations. Consider this: What if you take an antibiotic to treat an MRSA infection and it kills all of the dangerous bacteria, except for one single bacterium (bacterium is the singular form of bacteria). That one super-strong bacterium survives and multiplies, making more super-strong bacteria. All of the weaker bacteria have been killed, but now you have many, many super-strong bacteria that are likely to be resistant to the original antibiotic (and to other antibiotics as well).

SUPER BUGS LOVE HOSPITALS

Remember the old joke about banks:

Harry: "Why do people rob banks?"
Larry: "Because that's where the money is."

It's the same for super bugs. Why do hospitals have so many super bugs? Because that's where the sick people with infections are.

There are three reasons why MRSA, VRE, and *C. diff* have made hospitals their favorite home:

- A majority of hospitalized patients are given antibiotics, which increases the chance that "good" bacteria will be killed, while "bad" bacteria like *C. difficile* will survive and be passed on to other patients.
- People who are sick enough to need hospitalization often have weakened immune systems that can't fight infections, so they're more likely to catch any super bug that comes their way.
- Many healthcare workers don't wash their hands well enough or often enough. That means super bugs living anywhere in a hospital may be quickly transmitted from patient to patient, either on healthcare workers' hands or patients' bed rails, other surfaces in the patients' rooms, food trays, medical equipment, and more.

Studies show that transmission of MRSA, VRE, and *C. difficile* from one patient to another occurs mostly via the hands of healthcare workers. I have conducted observational studies of handwashing in numerous hospitals around the country, so I know for sure that healthcare workers wash or sanitize their hands less than 50 percent of the time.

ARE THERE ANY SAFE HOSPITALS?

When hospitals hire me to help improve their infection control, I always focus on ways to ensure that all healthcare workers and patients consistently wash and disinfect their hands. That can make a big difference!

But I know it's impossible to completely prevent super bug infections, especially in larger hospitals and in intensive care units (ICUs) where a high percentage of patients are gravely ill or very elderly. You may hear that you have a lower risk of super bug infections at most smaller hospitals and children's hospitals where patients are less likely to be severely ill, there's no guarantee. But keep in mind that the number of super bug infections is increasing, so hospital size may not be as important as we once believed. That's the reason you need to be on your guard to make sure healthcare workers wash their hands.

The TV Camera Was on But They Still Didn't Wash!

When I first began doing research and published my first article, many TV stations wanted to interview me about my method of having patients remind healthcare workers to wash their hands. I learned very quickly that the media usually adds a "twist" to the story, in addition to the ordinary facts.

So there I was in an intensive care unit with a national TV reporter questioning me about my research. Toward the end of the interview, he asked me to demonstrate the correct way people should wash their hands, while he continued to comment. An important note: I was amazed that the reporter made it very clear to me that he needed to stand on a certain side of the sink, because he wanted to be filmed only on his "good side." That did seem a little strange, but I still thought the interview went well.

On the night the report was scheduled for broadcast, I gathered my family around the TV with me to view my 15 minutes of fame. To my surprise, as soon as I began speaking to the reporter, two round clicking clocks appeared on the screen above me. One clock was set for 15 seconds, which is the recommended amount of time people need to wash their hands. The other clock started ticking whenever the screen showed a healthcare worker either begin to wash her hands or fail to wash in a situation where she should have. Yes, unbeknownst to me, someone from the TV station had used a hidden camera to record what all the ICU healthcare workers were doing.

You could say it's wrong not to disclose this secret filming, and that would be valid. But the real issue is that everyone taking care of the patients in the ICU could see that a TV reporter was filming an interview about hand hygiene. You might think everyone would be sure to do the correct thing. Well, much to our embarrassment, the film showed that in addition to those who did not wash at all, most healthcare workers who did wash their hands never did it for the full 15 seconds.

THE BUGS KEEP SPREADING

Cases of multidrug-resistant infection are steadily increasing everywhere in the United States and around the world, so it's hard for patients in any hospital to avoid exposure to super bugs. For example, in the early 1990s, there was only a 20–25 percent chance that a healthcare-associated *Staphylococcus* infection would be methicillin resistant. Today, there's a 60 percent chance that a similar *Staph* infection would be resistant. The most recent statistics from the U.S. Centers for Disease Control and Prevention show that 94,380 patients developed invasive MRSA infections in the United Sates in 2005; 18,850 of these patients died.[17]

Increasing outbreaks have also occurred with VRE infections, which have gone from a less than 1 percent chance of being antibiotic resistant in 1997 to an almost 30 percent chance in 2003. And for *C. diff*, the numbers have doubled from about 40 cases per 100,000 patients in the U.S. population in the 1990s to 84 cases per 100,000 in 2005. A study in England reported *C. diff* infection as the primary cause of death for 499 people in 1999, rising to 3,393 in 2006.[18]

MRSA, VRE, and *C. diff* are the most common super bugs. They're the ones you're most likely to hear about on TV and read about in newspapers and on the Internet. But these days, almost every month brings a report of new antibiotic-resistant bacteria. Look at the chart on page 33, which shows the steady increase in MRSA and VRE infections. You'll also notice a new super bug category, *Pseudomonas*, which first showed up around 1989. More recently in 2009, doctors reported a newer antibiotic-resistant bug, New Delhi metallo-beta-lactamase, named after the city in which a Swedish tourist contracted the first case.[19] As this indicates, infections are moving from country to country, so don't be surprised if next week's news headlines include yet another new super bug warning.

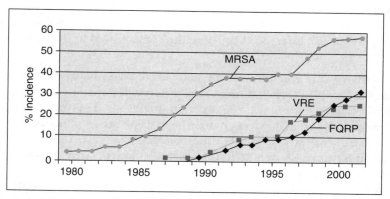

This chart shows the increase in rates of resistance for three bacteria that are of concern to public health officials; methicillin-resistant *Staphylococcus aureus* (MRSA), vancomycin-resistant enterococci (VRE), and fluoroquinolone-resistant *Pseudomonas aeruginosa* (FQRP). These data were collected from hospital intensive care units that participate in the National Nosocomial Infections Surveilance System, a component of the CDC. From the Centers for Disease Control and Prevention.

Q: Are some patients more likely to get an infection with multidrug-resistant bacteria?

A: Yes, super bug infections occur more often in people whose immune system defenses are weakened due to AIDS, cancer chemotherapy, recent surgery, and other medical conditions. Risk of infection is also higher for people using urinary catheters or ventilators and for those who have longer hospitalizations or require treatment in an intensive care unit.

Q: Why is there a high risk of infection in an intensive care unit? Aren't doctors and nurses especially careful there?

A: Patients in the ICU are very sick, which means they're more likely to have been infected with resistant bacteria before they went into the ICU. The more patients in the ICU at one time, the greater is the risk that an infected person's bacteria will be transmitted to other ICU patients. Although the sickest patients are in the ICU, multidrug-resistant bacteria are currently found in increasing numbers in non-ICU patients.

Q: Don't hospitals know which patients are infected, so those patients can be kept away from others?

A: Many people are colonized with bacteria on their skin or in their body, even if those bacteria haven't caused an infection yet. Although there are no signs of infection, people who are colonized can still transmit the bacteria to others. There lies the problem that prevents hospitals from finding out which patients are infected at the time they're admitted to the hospital.

Pennsylvania and a few other states have passed laws that require all patients to have bacterial cultures performed when they're admitted to the hospital as a check for multidrug-resistant infections. This makes it easier to take precautions that may decrease the risk of other patients becoming infected. Several studies in Europe, particularly research done in the Netherlands, have shown that this "search and destroy" approach can significantly decrease the incidence of super bug infections.[20]

Before you are admitted to a hospital, find out whether bacterial cultures are routinely performed on admission. If not, the most important thing you can do is to insist that doctors, nurses, and other healthcare workers always wash or sanitize their hands before and after they have contact with you.

HOW TO PROTECT YOURSELF IN THE HOSPITAL

It's frightening to think of everything that can go wrong when you are hospitalized. The purpose of this book is not to scare you, but instead to help you to protect yourself from infections and treatment errors, so you won't feel so frightened. There's nothing complicated about it, honestly! Here are some simple tips to remember:

- First, and most important, I'll repeat: Ask all healthcare workers to wash or sanitize their hands before they have contact with you.
- Make sure you practice what we call interventional patient hygiene, a fancy way to define bathing. This means that *you* control the bacteria that are on your skin by keeping your body clean. *You* decrease the possibility of super bugs getting into your system at the site of your surgical incision, or during insertion of an intravenous line, or when you are touched by healthcare workers, or when you come in contact with objects in your hospital room.
- Take precautions at bath time. Make sure you have a bath each day using prepackaged towels, preferably ones that have been treated with chlorhexidine to kill bacteria. Hospitals should provide these for you. Do not allow

yourself to be washed using a basin and towels. Basin water can be a source of bacteria. If you're told the safer technique isn't used, refuse the bath and ask a friend or family member to bring you a supply of pre-packaged towels and help you with bathing.

■ Finally, if you are in the Intensive Care Unit, or if you are unable to help yourself after surgery, be sure to have a family member or friend with you to act as an "advocate" who will request the care and precautions you need.

As you've read, there are numerous ways that improper use of antibiotics can contribute to a continued increase in the creation of super bugs. But you, the patient, can help to break this chain of transmission.

Q: Many people are routinely given antibiotics before or after surgery to prevent infections. Is this safe? Or is it dangerous overuse of antibiotics that could create resistant bacteria?

A: If your doctor says you need antibiotics before surgery (this is called surgical prophylaxis), the first thing you should do is to ask[21]:

- Is there any another treatment option instead of antibiotic use?
- Is presurgery antibiotic treatment the proven approach to preventing infections for the kind of surgery I'm having?
- Are you using an antibiotic with the narrowest spectrum for this purpose? That means choosing a drug that kills only the bacteria that are expected to be present and not a drug that kills a large selection of bacteria. Limiting the targets limits the risk of creating antibiotic resistance.
- When will the antibiotic be administered? Antibiotics for surgical prophylaxis usually should not be given for more than 24 hours. In most cases, postoperative doses are not required.
- Remember if you do not get answers or are told don't worry, find another surgeon.

Q: What should be done if I get an infection during my hospitalization?

A: First, doctors should be sure that it's a bacterial infection and not a viral or fungal infection before any antibiodics are given to you. Viral illnesses such as acute bronchitis should never be treated with antibiotics. Here's what to look for[17]:

- The key is to identify the pathogen—that is, for the doctor to take a tissue or fluid sample and send it to the laboratory for a culture that will reveal what kind of bacteria are present and which antibiotics they are most susceptible to.

- If your symptoms are easily identified as a bacterial infection, your doctor may decide to start antibiotic treatment before culture results are in. This is known as empiric therapy. It's important to receive empiric therapy that targets the pathogens that have been detected recently in your hospital and in the local area, or are the most frequently found bacteria for the body site of your surgery. Most hospitals have a "local biogram" that provides this information.
- When culture results come in, the empiric antibiotic should be replaced, if necessary, with the antibiotic that best matches your antimicrobial susceptibility test results. The doctor should select an antibiotic with the narrowest spectrum for the type of bacteria that was identified. This is known as definitive therapy.

While you're still hospitalized, be sure the antibiotic is given to you as often as the doctor has directed. If you know you should be taking a pill twice a day, and the nurse has not arrived with one of your doses, let the nurses know and have them check your chart to see when the last pill was administered. You must complete the recommended days of treatment. Do not skip a dosage or stop taking the antibiotic, even if you feel better. That can lead to growth of resistant bacteria.

Q. When should antibiotic treatment be stopped?[17]

A: If cultures that were taken when you were showing signs of infection come back negative and your symptoms suggest that infection is unlikely. When you have finished the antibiotic treatment and the infection is considered cured.

Take Your Antibiotic as Directed!

DO take your antibiotic as directed

DO finish all of your antibiotic

DO NOT skip a dose of your antibiotic

DO NOT take antibiotics for viral infections

DO NOT save your antibiotics for another time

DO NOT take another person's antibiotics

Q: What should I do if my infection symptoms get worse, despite antibiotic treatment?

A: Ask your doctor to consult with an infectious diseases expert. If there are no experts in your hospital, ask your doctors to arrange for an outside consult. If he/she refuses this would be a time for you or your advocate to request a rapid response as discussed in Chapter 1. You could have an antibiotic-resistant infection, so getting expert advice on which antibiotic or other treatment to use could save you from major complications or even death.

Q: What should I do if I think I'm developing an infection after I'm home from the hospital?

A: As you've read before, bacterial colonization can take considerable time to turn into actual infection. With super bugs, symptoms of infection typically develop while a patient is still hospitalized. But in some cases, symptoms may appear weeks or even months after hospitalization. If that happens to you, be sure to tell your doctor that you have been hospitalized recently and whether you have received antibiotic therapy.

Q: What infection symptoms should I look for?

A: Whether you're in the hospital or back at home, you could have an infection if you're experiencing chills or fever, unexpected pain, drainage or pus oozing from a wound site, or increased inflammation of a surgical incision. If any of these symptoms occur, call your doctor immediately, especially if you have recently been discharged from a hospital.

WHEN MRSA STRIKES

This chapter is full of facts about dangerous super bug infections. To me, what really brings these facts to life are the many stories I hear from people who have generously shared their stories like Carrie Simon who has "been there" and lived to tell the tale. Here's the story in Carrie's own words:

Why didn't anyone tell me about MRSA? My name is Carrie Simon. I had never heard of methicillin-resistant *Staphylococcus aureus* (MRSA) before I was infected with it. This is quite surprising, because I have been in and out of hospitals for most of my adult life. My story begins when I was 17 and was diagnosed with Hodgkin's disease, cancer of the lymphatic system (a rare lymphoma). That was 33 years ago. Here I am today: a wife, a mother of three teenage daughters, and a teacher. And on top of that, I am actively involved in my continuing survival!

The long-term effects of radiation treatment have given me severe medical problems, including cardiac disease that affects the valves of my heart . . . I was under the care of experts in the long-term effects of cancer survivorship . . . who put me in contact with a cardiologist at a large academic medical center in a major city. I felt very good about the care that I would receive.

After listening to that doctor's best advice, I underwent an aortic valve replacement and tricuspid and mitral valve repairs. As we all expected, the surgery went very well, but a few days later . . . my pain gradually began to increase instead of decrease. Neither the nursing staff nor the resident physicians recognized the significance of my symptoms. Only after about 36 hours of an unexplainable deterioration in my condition, and the onset of near-fatal atrial fibrillation, did the hospital staff respond appropriately. . . . I was rushed from the step-down unit back to the intensive care unit.

I clearly remember the painful day when the infectious disease doctor told me that he thought I had contracted a life-threatening antibiotic-resistant MRSA infection that was ravaging my body. . . . As a result, I underwent *five additional* surgeries during which a cardiac surgeon debrided my sternum (that is, scraped away infected tissue from my breastbone) and disinfected my chest wound.

I remained hospitalized for more than 2 months. During that time, I sank into a deep depression. My family arranged for a psychiatrist to visit me each day, but nothing could change the reality of my situation. My oldest daughter was in her first year of college in New York, my other two children were in school in Connecticut, and I was in a hospital in Boston. My children were terrified, and I was helpless.

We did not know whether treatment with intravenous vancomycin (an antibiotic) would work. I vomited from that therapy every day. In addition, I experienced drainage complications as result of the current surgeries and past radiation therapy, so the days just dragged on.

My family and friends helped me through this crisis. All the while I was in Boston, I was never alone. My husband, parents, cousin, and friends were there with me. They were my constant companions, but more importantly, they were my advocates. Thrust into a life-threatening challenge, my husband began to research this "mysterious" infectious disease. Many of the hospital physicians were loathe to communicate about it with me, but it was obvious that I was not the only patient with an MRSA infection in the cardiac intensive care unit.

As a practicing attorney, my husband used his research skills to learn all he could about MRSA and how it had quietly developed into an epidemic problem in U.S. hospitals. *How could this infection, which was affecting so many cardiac patients at a nationally recognized teaching hospital, not have been the subject of our preoperative discussions? How could the medical staff, including highly acclaimed cardiac fellows, have been so unaware of the obvious signs of that infection that developed?* Those questions undermined our confidence in a hospital that we had carefully chosen as the place to minimize the risks that surgery entailed for me as a Hodgkin's disease survivor.

After I had been hospitalized for 9 weeks, my condition had improved. Although my doctors did not think that I was ready to leave, I could not stand it there any longer. I was still depressed, and I was unable to eat because of nausea caused by the antibiotic therapy. I insisted that I be allowed to go home.

After I returned home, my emotional state gradually improved, and I began to eat again. I received medical care from visiting nurses, and my husband was in charge of administering 6 additional weeks of intravenous vancomycin. My health gradually improved, too, but the emotional scars have taken their toll on my family, my friends, and me.

As a Hodgkin's disease survivor, I know that I will need to be hospitalized from time to time to deal with the long-term effects of my illness. Since my cardiac surgery and the subsequent MRSA complications that I experienced 2 years ago, I have been hospitalized 4 times: once for breast cancer, twice for unexplained bleeding in my gastrointestinal system, and once to have a pacemaker implanted. Each time I entered the hospital, I was terrified that I would contract a MRSA infection again. Thankfully, I was fortunate each of those times.

Carrie Simon's memorable story paints a vivid picture of how devastating super bug infections can be. But on the positive side, she also reveals how a patient and family and friends can play an active part in demanding the attention and care that's vitally needed. The checklist at the end of the chapter is a quick reminder of easy steps you can take to help yourself or a loved one who is hospitalized.

WE WILL REACH OUR GOAL!

My work over the past 6 years involves collecting data from hospitals across the United States from which I determine their hand hygiene "compliance rate" every month. By compliance, I mean: Do healthcare workers actually wash or sanitize their hands every time hand hygiene is required? The bad news is that the average compliance rate in intensive care units is only 26 percent. In non-ICU units, compliance averages 37 percent. The good news is that when hospitals educate their patients to ask healthcare workers to wash and sanitize their hands, we've found that hand hygiene compliance increases to 37 percent in the ICU and 51 percent in non-ICU units.[22] That's still not great, but it's definitely an improvement. The more patients who start asking healthcare professionals to wash their hands, the closer we'll get to our goal of 100 percent hand hygiene compliance.

Did you know that if you are a patient in an intensive care unit, all the healthcare workers involved in your care will have a total of 144 times when they should perform hand hygiene during each 24 hour period? That's 6 times every hour. If you are in a non-ICU room, the total would be 72 times every 24 hours. With so many chances to forget during a busy day caring for patients, it's no wonder that nurses' and doctors' hand hygiene rates are so low.

So if you wind up in a hospital bed, start counting and start asking. Healthcare workers need your help!

Remember, when hospitalized . . .

1. When hospitalized, make sure you have a daily bath.
2. Tell all healthcare workers and visitors to wash or sanitize their hands.
3. Tell your doctor if you have recently been: hospitalized, admitted to a nursing home, exposed to or treated for MRSA, or currently have an infection (for example, urinary tract).
4. Identify an advocate and understand the use of "rapid response."
5. Discuss informed consent and ask your surgeon about infection rates and antibiotics.
6. Check your skin around an IV for any redness or swelling.
7. Urinary catheters should only be used when necessary, not for convenience.
8. After discharge, check your wound site for any redness, swelling, or drainage, if you have pain.

© *MMI, Inc.* 2004, Ardmore, PA; www.hhreports.com

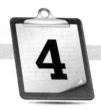

Let's Talk Dirty:
Hand Hygiene
and
Patient Hygiene

Stop what you're doing—right now!

Your hands are dirty, and I need you to go wash them right away.

You say you just washed them? Wash them again!

Trust me—I'm a handwashing expert. I'm *sure* your hands are still dirty.

Go wash them again and then come back.

THE DIRTY TRUTH

Back already? Let's check to see if you did a good job.

Hold up your hands and move them like the hands you see in the figure that follows.

HAND HYGIENE TECHNIQUE WITH SOAP AND WATER

🕐 **Duration of the entire procedure: 40-60 seconds**

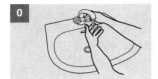

Wet hands with water

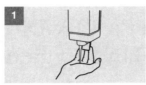

Apply enough soap to cover all hand surface

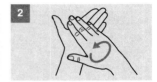

Rub hands palm to palm

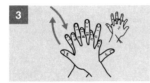

Right palm over left dorsum with interlaced fingers and vice versa

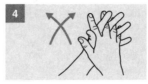

Palm to palm with fingers interlaced

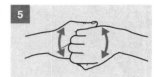

Backs of fingers to opposing palms with fingers interlocked

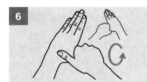

Rotational rubbing of left thumb clasped in right palm and vice versa

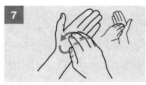

Rotational rubbing, backward and forward with clasped fingers of right hand in left palm and vice versa

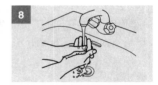

Rinse hands with water

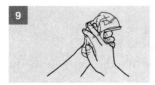

Dry hands throughly with a single use towel

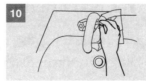

Use towel to turn off faucet

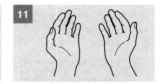

Your hands are now safe.

How to hand wash (11 steps).

(WHO Guidelines on Hand Hygiene in Healthcare. WHO, 2009.)

Missed Spots

When you were washing, I bet you did fine on steps 0, 1, 2, and 8, but I'd be surprised if you washed by interlacing or interlocking your fingers (steps 3, 4, and 5). Did you also leave out rubbing your palms with clasped fingers (steps 6 and 7)? Your hands may look clean without doing all this, but your eyes can't spot the microscopic germs you left behind. Look at the drawing below, and you'll see what you probably missed.

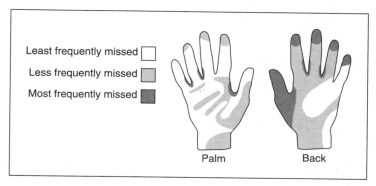

Areas of the hands most frequently missed during handwashing.
(Adapted from Manchester NHS North, Central, and South Primary Care Hand Hygiene Guidelines, April 2005.)

Most people spend 15 seconds or less washing their hands, because they skip steps 3, 4, 5, 6, and 7, and rush through 1, 2, 8, and 9. If you perform all 11 recommended handwashing steps, the whole process would probably take about 40-60 seconds. Trained healthcare workers who wash their hands in between patients many times a day can often do a satisfactory job in 15-20 seconds. But as you know, many doctors and nurses speed through carelessly, even when TV cameras are watching.

Hand Sanitizing

If you're in a rush and don't want to spend even 40 seconds, you can achieve good results in about 20-30 seconds by using a hand sanitizer—but only if your hands aren't visibly dirty. (You need soap to remove visible dirt.) As you can see in the following diagram, steps 2 through 7 are the same for hand sanitizer cleansing as with handwashing, but there's no need for rinsing and drying.

HAND HYGIENE TECHNIQUE WITH HAND SANITIZER

🕐 **Duration of the entire procedure: 20-30 seconds**

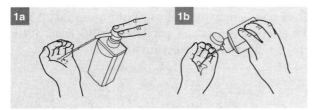

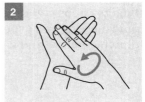

Apply a palmful of the product in a cupped hand, covering all surfaces

Rub hands palm to palm

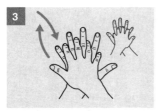

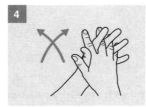

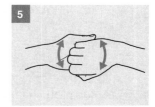

Right palm over left dorsum with interlaced fingers and vice versa

Palm to palm with fingers interlaced

Backs of fingers to oppposing palms with fingers interlocked

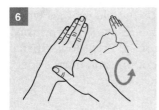

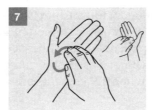

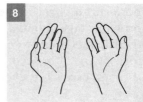

Rotational rubbing of left thumb clasped in right palm and vice versa

Rotational rubbing, backward and forward with clasped fingers of right hand in left palm and vice versa

Once dry, your hands are safe.

How to use a hand sanitizer.
(WHO Guidelines on Hand Hygiene in Healthcare, 2009.)

Try it again! Many restrooms don't provide hand sanitizers, so let's assume that your hands are visibly dirty right now and you need to wash them. Please take this book over to the sink with you and wash your hands again. This time, try not to skip any of the 11 steps.

Finished? How did it go? It wasn't very difficult, was it?

Actually, handwashing is pretty simple. However, most people were never taught how to do it right when they were children, or they weren't taught that it's really important. A study about kids and handwashing that I did with my daughter, Maryellen, when she was in middle school bears this out.[1] By the way, it won a first prize at a science forum and was published in a journal. Maryellen, with the help of her brother, monitored bathrooms in the middle school and high school divisions of two single-sex private schools (60 boys and 60 girls, total). They disguised their purpose by pretending to wait to use the sink area, while they watched to see how many students washed their hands.

What do you think they found? During a 4-week period, only 48 percent of male students washed their hands after bathroom use, compared with 58 percent of female students. Even worse news: Only 8 percent of the boys and 28 percent of the girls used soap when they washed, and a majority of all students washed for less than 5 seconds. Would you want to shake hands with any of those kids?

And don't think it's just children. In a similar study of adults using public restrooms at a large railroad station, observers found that only 60 percent of people washed up afterward.[2] Think about it: Do you *always* wash your hands when you use a public bathroom? Or at home after using the toilet? Or before and after preparing food? Now look back to the diagram of frequently missed areas on the hands on page 45. I hope you'll decide that 40 seconds of handwashing is well worth your time and effort.

THE GREAT UNWASHED

If handwashing is important for ordinary people, consider how much more important it is for doctors, nurses, and other healthcare workers who come in contact with sick patients. Just by touching a patient's hand or shoulder or taking the patient's pulse, doctors and other healthcare workers can pick up dangerous bacteria on their hands that, for their own protection, they'd certainly want to wash away. Of course, washing is also important to prevent all healthcare workers from passing one patient's bacteria on to other patients and onto bedrails, tables, walls, and other surfaces in patients' rooms and throughout the hospital.

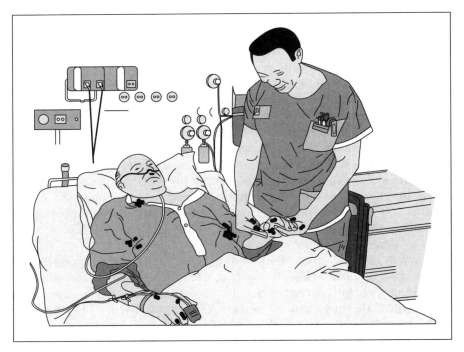

Bacteria transfer from patient to healthcare worker's hands.
Contact between the healthcare worker and the patient results in cross-transmission of microorganisms. In this case, Gram-positive cocci from the patient's own flora transfer tohealthcare worker's hands.
Reprinted from Pittet, 2006 with permission from Elsevier.

Even if your parents never taught you the right way to wash your hands, I guarantee you that doctors, nurses, and most other healthcare workers have been taught the proper procedure. Unfortunately, they're often too rushed, or too forgetful, to do any better than you just did. We know from several hand hygiene studies that less than 50 percent of healthcare workers wash their hands before touching patients—and some studies have shown that it's only 20–30 percent.[3]

As you just found by trying it, there's a big difference between washing and washing correctly. During my hospital studies, I saw that even when healthcare workers do remember to wash, it's typically for a shorter time than is recommended. This is not safe. In fact, in one of our studies, we actually found that people in an airport restroom washed their hands longer than people who worked in a hospital's intensive care unit![4]

Thorough handwashing is so important for healthcare workers that the World Health Organization has issued a 300-page set of guidelines covering all aspects of hand hygiene that workers must follow to protect patients.[5] Of course, the guidelines include all of the handwashing and hand sanitizing steps shown in the diagrams in this chapter, along with the requirement that healthcare workers must cleanse their hands *before* and *after* contact with each patient.

Even small details are included in the WHO guidelines. For example, because bacteria collect under the fingernails, workers should trim their fingernails to less than a quarter of an inch and should not use artificial and extended nails. Healthcare workers must also remove watches, rings, and other bacteria-trapping jewelry and roll up their sleeves to permit washing the lower one-third of their arms. (Apart from WHO, some experts also wonder whether doctors' neckties should be banned, because the tail ends may touch patients during an examination,[6] and whether stethoscopes need frequent antibacterial cleaning.[7,8])

Attention to all these patient safety measures is making a real difference in hospital safety. For example, hospitals that are using a hygiene program developed by the Joint Commission, which also works with WHO, increased their rate of handwashing and sanitizing from an average of 48 percent in April 2009, to 82 percent in less than a year.[9]

Q: Why don't healthcare workers always wash or sanitize their hands?

A: When I asked that question in my surveys, healthcare workers' top three reasons for not washing their hands were: (1) "My hands get red and crack when I wash too often," (2) "I wear gloves instead," and (3) "I forget."

Q: Is there really a big risk that I could get an infection just because a doctor or nurse touches me without first washing his hands?

A: In many hospitals, healthcare workers still wash their hands less than 50 percent of the time after they have touched something or someone. This means that every time a doctor, nurse, technician, food server, or anyone else in a hospital touches a hospital surface or another person and then touches you, you have a 50 percent chance of getting bacteria from their hands.

Q: Does a healthcare worker need to do anything else besides wash his or her hands in order to prevent my getting an infection from drug-resistant bacteria like methicillin-resistant *Staphylococcus aureus* (MRSA) while I'm in the hospital?

A: Thorough cleaning of patients' rooms and the entire hospital building and prescribing antibiotics only when necessary are two things that can help, but the simplest and most effective single action is hand hygiene.

Q: Do medical personnel always need to use soap and water to clean their hands before they touch me?

A: No. Healthcare workers should use soap and water only if their hands are dirty with blood or other body fluids. Otherwise, we now recommend that they can use a hand sanitizer. Sanitizers are waterless products (most contain alcohol) that work better than soap and water at killing bacteria and viruses. They're also gentler to the hands, which is very helpful for medical personnel who must wash their hands numerous times a day. Sanitizers are usually found in a dispenser on the wall in each hospital room or outside the room.

Q: Should I use the sanitizer in my hospital room to sanitize my own hands?

A: Yes. It is important that patients also sanitize or wash their hands. Bacteria can live for days on surfaces that you will touch (such as bed railings and doorknobs), so washing or sanitizing your hands will prevent you from infecting yourself with bacteria or viruses. Also be sure to wash your hands after you use the bathroom or a bedpan, or when you have been in another part of the hospital and then return to your room. Some hospitals give people a small bottle of sanitizer to use during their stay. Showing your healthcare workers your bottle of sanitizer is a good way of reminding them to wash and/or sanitize their hands.

TAKE FIVE TO STAY ALIVE!

You've just finished reading about the many steps that healthcare workers must follow when they wash or sanitize their hands. It's important for you to know *how* they should do it, but you also need to know *when* they absolutely, positively, must wash or sanitize their hands. By knowing that, you'll know when you, as a patient, should watch to see that healthcare workers are washing or sanitizing their hands.

Many hospitals face a shortage of doctors, nurses, and other medical personnel, so it's not surprising that extremely busy healthcare workers sometimes forget hand-washing. To simplify workers' tasks, the experts who formulated the World Health Organization Hand Hygiene Guidelines identified the five most crucial situations ("moments") in which medical personnel absolutely, positively MUST wash or sanitize their hands.[10]

Look at the drawing below. Now imagine yourself as the patient in that bed. What should you be watching for?

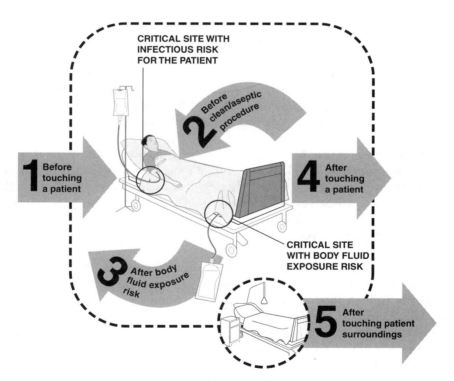

Your five moments for hand hygiene.
Hand hygiene must be performed as described, whether gloves are used or not.
(WHO Hand Hygiene: Why, How & When? Brochure, revised August 2009.)

Moment 1: Is a healthcare worker or a guest about to enter your room? It could be a doctor or nurse coming in to take your pulse or blood pressure, listen to your heart, give you a bath, or even stroke your arm as a friendly gesture of comfort. That's when medical personnel and everyone else should wash or sanitize their hands before making any contact with you.

Moment 2: Will a healthcare worker come in contact with mucous membranes in your mouth (for oral or dental care), your eyes (administering eye drops), or openings in your skin (for wound cleaning, insertion of a catheter, or changing a drain device)? Hand hygiene is crucial before any of these aseptic ("clean") procedures.

Moment 3: It describes the situations in which healthcare workers obtain blood or urine samples from you, clean up urine or feces, or dispose of used bandages, incontinence pads, and other waste. The worker must clean her hands immediately after such an exposure to protect you and the surrounding area from harmful bacteria. If the worker was wearing gloves, the worker must wash her hands after removing the gloves. (More on glove use is coming up.)

Moment 4: It is a follow-up to Moment 1. Handwashing is important before someone touched you, but it's equally important afterward. Whenever healthcare workers leave your bedside after working with you, watch to be sure that they wash their hands. This protects you and the entire hospital from any harmful germs that may have been transmitted from your body.

Moment 5: It is something many healthcare workers and patients hardly think about: germ transmission from objects in the room. Even though food delivery people, linen changing staff, and cleaning workers may not even put a finger on you, their hands are coming in contact with your bed rail, night table, food table, food tray, and any equipment they may need to adjust. All these people and anyone else who is about to enter your room should use the hand sanitizer dispenser mounted near the doorway to kill germs on their hands before they come in. Stop anyone from carrying dirty linens or other contaminated items *into* your room, and if necessary, remind people to wash their hands when going *out* of your room or coming back in.

Q: If I'm a patient, is there anything I can do to ensure that my healthcare workers wash or sanitize their hands for each of the five moments?

A: Yes. As we'll talk about in the next chapter, it's up to you to remind healthcare workers about hand-washing. You can do this just by saying, "Could you please wash or sanitize your hands?" If you are hospitalized, you are the only person who is in that hospital bed all the time, so you are the only one who can constantly prompt healthcare workers about hand-washing. If family members or friends come by to help you, tell them to wash or sanitize their hands, and to make hand-washing reminders, too.

Q: Will healthcare workers get mad at me for reminding them about hand-washing?

A: Some may, but some will thank you. As I mentioned above, one of the top three reasons that healthcare workers don't wash their hands is that they "forget." Your reminder is actually helping them not to forget to wash or sanitize their hands.

Because hospital-associated infections are expensive to treat, hospitals urgently want to prevent them. By reminding healthcare workers about correct hand hygiene, you'll be helping the hospital, too, as well as protecting yourself from illness.

Q: What should I do if my healthcare worker refuses to wash or sanitize his or her hands?

A: There is only one response for this: You must *insist* that the healthcare workers washes or sanitizes his or her hands.

Don't be shy! Bacteria and infections know no boundaries. Don't assume that it's OK to skip hand-washing occasionally. It's not. The one time that you don't remind a healthcare worker to wash his or her hands could very well be the time that you acquire a potentially fatal MRSA super bug infection.

If you can't persuade a worker to wash or sanitize, stop everything and ask to speak with the nursing supervisor for your unit, or immediately telephone your hospital's patient advocate or rapid response team. The booklet or patient information print out you received when you were admitted to the hospital always includes this emergency phone number. I can assure you that your healthcare workers will comply when you let them know that you are aware of this complaint process.

Remember: One patient, one healthcare worker, one question: Did you wash and/or sanitize your hands?

Make sure that any physician, nurse, therapist, or other healthcare worker has washed his or her hands before touching you.

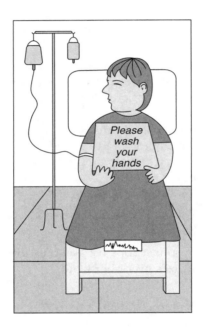

Meet the Glove Brigade

Seeing a doctor or nurse put on sterile gloves gives people a false sense of security. Do not feel protected if a healthcare worker merely puts on gloves before examining or treating you. Did he first wash or sanitize his hands?

You could certainly assume that unused medical gloves taken out of a fresh box or a sterile wrapper are truly clean, but you're probably wrong,

Even if the person who takes them out has washed his or her hands thoroughly, bacteria that are left on the hands immediately migrate onto and into the gloves. And what if the wearer's sharp nails caused a tiny hole that's invisible to the eye but quite large enough for millions of bacteria to sneak through?

It gets worse than that. Bacteria multiply quickly in a moist environment like the inside of a glove. Because bacteria reproduce every 20 minutes, a healthcare worker who didn't wash his hands thoroughly before donning the gloves will have millions of bacteria on his or her hands when the gloves come off. If that worker then puts on a new pair of gloves without first washing or using hand sanitizer, those new gloves will also be contaminated on the outside and the inside.

Imagine that this careless healthcare worker arrives at your hospital room wearing those same gloves. Just seeing his gloved hands gives you confidence that you'll be protected from germs while the worker examines you. Of course, that's only because you know nothing about where's he's been and what he's done with those gloves before you saw him. Now imagine that he goes first to help the patient in bed 1, acquiring more bacteria on his gloves and not changing the gloves and washing his hands. Uh oh! He's approaching your bed! Are you still feeling confident about this gloved one?

Misconceptions About Gloves

This tale is just imaginary, but numerous studies done by me and many others have shown that misuse of gloves is rampant in hospitals everywhere.[9] My concern is that the new hand-washing and sanitizing guidelines from WHO, the Joint Commission, and the U.S. Centers for Disease Control and Prevention are not being followed and in fact have simply been replaced by the use of gloves as an alternative to hand hygiene. I'm also concerned about healthcare workers' frequent misconception that gloves are for *their* protection, not the patient's.

Let me give you an example of something I observed in an intensive care unit, of all places. A nurse enters the room, goes directly to the box of gloves, puts on gloves, and then passes the sink and the hand sanitizer. She proceeds to the patient to insert an intravenous line, wearing the same gloves. When I questioned her about not having removed the gloves and sanitizing her hands before contact with the patient, she had a look of confusion, protesting that her gloves were not torn or soiled.

Gloves *Do* Help

Of course, gloves do play an important role in many medical situations and often help to prevent many types of healthcare-associated infections. For example, the Centers for Disease Control and Prevention recommends that healthcare workers put on clean gloves (nonsterile ones are okay) when they anticipate contact with contaminated items or surfaces, blood, mucous membranes, nonintact skin, or intact skin that might have been exposed to feces or urine.

In some situations, gloves are actually a good second defense after handwashing or hand sanitizer use. Remember what you read about *C. difficile* super bugs? Even though handwashing can help to eliminate *C. difficile* spores, studies show that wearing gloves is significantly more effective in reducing the transmission of *C. difficile* super bug infection.[5] On the other hand, vancomycin-resistant enterococci (VRE) were found to stick to gloved hands more than bare hands, so gloves aren't recommended for preventing VRE super bug infections.[11]

Medical gloves are meant for only one use. The same pair of gloves should not be used for the care of more than one patient in succession. As you've read, gloves should be removed after contact with a patient or other sources of contamination, and the wearer should immediately wash her hands.[12]

DON'T FORGET PATIENT HYGIENE

With all the attention to hand hygiene, let's not forget that the patient has a whole body to be concerned about. I tell hospital personnel to emphasize what's known as interventional patient hygiene—that is, procedures directly focused on fortifying patients' infection defenses through oral care, skin cleansing, and incontinence management.[13]

Get Bathed

That's where bathing comes in. We know that after 48 hours of being in a hospital, patients have acquired numerous bacteria by touching surfaces that are contaminated and by being in contact with healthcare workers who do not wash their hands. Unfortunately, because of personnel shortages, the hospital staff doesn't always get to bathing patients; the task is often left to family members. Remember in the last chapter I discussed the need to remind healthcare workers about your bathing routine, and I also discussed using chlorhexidine towels instead of soap and water for your bathing needs. You must address these bathing issues with the healthcare team. Studies show that when patients are bathed every day, the number of patients who acquire infections from MRSA and other drug-resistant bacteria do decrease. In Chapter 8, I'll tell you about other patient hygiene steps that should be performed before you have surgery to help prevent infections.

Cleaner Rooms

Environmental hygiene is important, too. You've read how contaminated surfaces spread bacteria from patient to patient and from healthcare workers to patients. Many studies have shown that careful cleaning of environmental surfaces in patients' rooms reduces infections.

To save money, many hospitals have reduced their cleaning crews. As a result, researchers find that hospital rooms are often not thoroughly cleaned after patients are discharged and before a new patient moves in. Consider what might happen if the prior occupant of your hospital bed was a person who had just died from MRSA.[14] I think you'll agree that cutting back on hospital cleaning is penny wise and pound foolish.

One more thing. You need to remember that the majority of patients leave the hospital infection free and feeling better than when they came in. In the next chapter, I'll give you many suggestions on active steps that you can take to make sure your next hospital stay ends just that way.

Don't Worry Too Much!

Please don't worry too much! Remember that the majority of patients leave the hospital infection free and feeling better than when they came in.

THINK TWICE ABOUT YOUR ROOMMATE AND YOUR HOSPITAL

I'm often called in as an expert witness to help people who have been harmed by serious hospital-associated infections. One of my most memorable cases involved "Mr. B.," a 72-year-old man whose right knee was so painfully stiff that it interfered with his golf game. He decided to have knee replacement surgery at a local hospital.

The replacement surgery went well. After a week's stay, Mr. B. was discharged in good shape. But one week later, the knee had become so infected that he had to be rehospitalized to have the knee drained. One month later, he again was readmitted for another knee drainage procedure. Seven months later, doctors found that the ongoing infection was eating away at Mr. B.'s bone. He was again hospitalized, this time to have the knee replacement removed.

The cultures of tissue removed from Mr. B.'s knee showed that his infection was caused by *Staph* bacteria, and also by *Klebseilla* and *Enterobacter*, both of which are found in the intestinal tract. How did this happen? Simply stated, "Someone did not wash their hands." How do I know this? Mr. B. had hired a lawyer to sue the hospital, and the lawyer called me in to investigate.

I put on my imaginary Sherlock Holmes hat and carefully reviewed Mr. B.'s hospital charts. What I found was not good. Check these clues for yourself:

1. Mr. B.'s roommate was a paraplegic. Such patients often get urinary tract infections. Indeed, his roommate had a urinary tract infection involving two bacteria. These bacteria were the same as those cultured from Mr. B.'s infected knee.
2. When I looked at the records of all the infections that had occurred in this hospital, I found that the hospital had a 30 percent increase in infections in the year Mr. B. had knee surgery.
3. When I questioned Mr. B.'s family about his initial hospital stay, they told me that they had seen his nurse not wash her hands before changing Mr. B.'s dressings. In fact, they reported that the same nurse once took a roll of gauze lying on the windowsill to use on his open wound. Obviously, these actions did not qualify as sterile technique.

It was clear to me that this hospital was responsible for Mr. B.'s infection, and that the single most important contributing factor was that the staff was not compliant in handwashing. As you saw, Mr. B. got the same type of infection as his roommate. Most likely, the room became contaminated with the roommate's bacteria. When healthcare workers failed to wash their hands and used contaminated medical supplies, bacteria in the room were transmitted to Mr. B.

You don't have to be Sherlock Holmes to guess the legal outcome: Mr. B. won the case.

Now that you're an experienced infection detective, use the Infection Prevention Checklist that follows to see what you should do if you're ever in a situation like Mr. B.'s. Remember, not all infections can be prevented, but infections like Mr. B.'s should never have occurred.

Infection Prevention Checklist

Going to the hospital?

1. Ask in advance about your hospital's infection rates. Are they going up?
2. Demand to be put in a room that's not shared by an infected patient. However, two patients with the same infection may, after evaluation, be put in same room.
3. Ask your healthcare workers to wash and sanitize their hands.
4. Tell your family that they must watch out for your needs when they're with you in the hospital. In their role as your "advocate" (a legal word for "spokesperson"), they must speak up if doctors, nurses, and other workers who are going to have direct contact with you have not properly cleaned their hands.

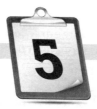

Power to the Patient

When you need hospital care, it's comforting to know that you've chosen a good hospital and a good doctor who will look out for your welfare. However, that doesn't mean you can just lie back and wait to get better. Whether you're in the hospital or back at home, you have definite rights and responsibilities for ensuring your own recovery.

But first, a word of caution. When you're admitted to the hospital and escorted to your room, you're entering a different universe. Depending on your medical insurance policy and your budget, you may find yourself sharing that room with one, two, three, or more other patients, whose TV choices, visitors, personal habits, and medical needs will intrude on your waking and sleeping hours. So much for privacy.

Settle in, take off your street clothes and put on the uniform that's given to you. It's the same awkward, open-in-the-back hospital gown everyone around you will be wearing. So much for style and individuality. Now get into your hospital bed, an industrial-style device that's higher, firmer, narrower, and probably less comfortable than the bed you've got at home. Don't be surprised if an aide puts the bedrails up, like a crib, so you won't fall out. You say you'd prefer a feather pillow? Sorry, no choices here. You can't sleep unless the room is dark? Sorry again, bright room lights are on all day and dim lights at night, so doctors, nurses, and aides can attend to patients—yourself included—at all hours.

You like to have dinner at 7 p.m.? Not at this establishment. Everyone here gets dinner at 5 p.m., breakfast at 7 a.m., and lunch at 11 a.m. And forget about sleeping 'til 8 or 9 a.m. Nursing shifts change at 7 a.m, so you'll be awakened before the night shift nurse leaves—perhaps even at 5:30 a.m. You're up too early and feeling lonely? You'll have to wait until 1 p.m. for visiting hours to start.

IT COULD HAPPEN TO YOU!

As you can see, hospitals encourage patients to submit without question to routines and medical procedures, including those that don't make much sense. Loss of individuality, lack of privacy, constant observation, and strict schedules can turn even the most assertive person into a passive captive.

Consider this story credited to the late Dr. Eda LeShan, a psychologist, author, radio and TV commentator: Dr. LeShan's good friend, "Mrs. Cooper," was hospitalized after a heart attack. Numerous wires and tubes tethered her to electronic machines that clicked and beeped continuously, while squiggly lines moved rapidly across a green TV monitor. One afternoon, everything suddenly fell silent. A nurse raced in, pushing a cart filled with medicine vials and equipment, while urging an aide to "Call a code!" When Mrs. Cooper protested, noting that she was talking, drinking juice, and apparently very much alive, the nurse shouted at her, "You can't be! Your heart has stopped beating!" The idea that the machines could be at fault, struck the nurse as ridiculous. But soon an electrician arrived, jiggled a few wires, and the monitors again started clicking.

Many hospitalized patients become so passive, weak, and frightened that they might indeed be convinced they're dead when machines stop working. I don't want that to happen to you! I'm about to turn you into an empowered patient, so you can get the hospital care you need and help to protect yourself from unintentional errors. You may be sick, but where your health is concerned, you're still in charge.

A NEW IDEA

Look up the word "power" in any dictionary and you'll see it defined as authority, control, clout, and strength. Definitely not words you'd use to describe actions of most hospital patients. But put the prefix "em" in front of "power" and that's a different story. When I *em*power you, I am giving you the information and tools you need to assert your authority, clout, and strength, so you can help to control what happens to you in the hospital.

What Is Empowerment?

In formal terms, empowerment has been defined as a process in which patients understand their opportunity to contribute, and are given the knowledge and skills by their healthcare provider and other educational sources to perform a task in an environment that recognizes community and cultural differences and encourages patient participation.[1]

Empowerment means gaining the knowledge, skills, and confidence you need to make choices and become an active participant in your healthcare.[2]

Today, we hear words like "empowerment," "involvement," "engagement," and "advocate"—all of which express the same goals to inform patients about their healthcare, about their choices, and about their role in preventing medical errors. Actually, patient empowerment is a relatively new idea. If you're a senior citizen, you probably remember popular hospital shows on TV in the 1960s, where the handsome young doctor, James Kildare (heartthrob actor Richard Chamberlain) confidently and caringly cured all his patients in just one hour. Or perhaps you preferred the more mature Marcus Welby, M.D., played by Robert Young in the same kindly, authoritative manner as in his TV role of *Father Knows Best*. With Dr. Kildare or Dr. Welby at their bedside, patients were content to follow these paternalistic doctors' orders without question.

You Gen X, Gen Y, and Echo Boomers in the Millennial Generation probably think of doctors and hospitals very differently, more like those in the *Dr. Oz* or *House* TV shows.

These two 21st-century doctors have more advanced medications, procedures, and equipment at their disposal than their 20th-century counterparts, but they're often busier and more rushed, due to insurance limitations and money-saving staff cutbacks. So, whether your doctor is more like Kildare and Welby or Oz or House, you really must be vigilant and knowledgeable to protect your welfare as a hospital patient. By doing this you will then understand why I say empowerment is a win–win strategy.[3]

THE 3 Cs OF EMPOWERMENT

Here's proof that you do need to be watchful. In 1999, the Institute of Medicine's division of the National Academy of Sciences reported that medical errors were causing almost 100,000 deaths and 1 million injuries each year in the United States.[4] These alarming findings increased public awareness and anger about hospital risks. In response, the Institute of Medicine set an ambitious goal of reducing harm to patients by 50 percent during the following 5 years.

That goal has not been met. In 2003, researchers reviewed medical records for over 6,000 people living in 12 metropolitan areas of the United States. They found that study participants had received only about 55 percent of the tests, medications, physical examinations, surgical procedures, and other recommended care that were required for their medical conditons.[5]

Little Improvement

More recently, a 2010 survey of over 2,000 patients admitted to North Carolina hospitals showed that harmful events are still common, with little evidence of any improvement.[6] During 2002–2007, about 18 percent of surveyed patients suffered harm during their hospital stay, mostly attributable to healthcare workers' failure to follow accepted safety procedures. Over 60 percent of these complications were judged to be preventable. Many required additional treatments and added days of hospitalization.

The two most commonly reported problems were (1) complications from medical procedures or medications and (2) healthcare-associated infections, such as urinary tract infections, surgical site infections, pneumonia, and infections from catheters in arteries and veins.

The Top Three Ways

How exactly can you become involved and empowered as an active participant in your healthcare team? Here are my top three ways—I've called them the "3 Cs" to help you remember them:

Commitment—You have an important stake (a personal investment) in your health, so you must commit to protecting it.

Continuity—You are the only person who is in the hospital room continuously, all the time, to make certain that your healthcare is performed correctly.

Communication—If you see something or need something, say something! Your healthcare workers can't guess what you're thinking and what help you may need.

Commitment, continuity, and communication are just a beginning. Taking action comes next. That will require:

- Careful attention to details of your care
- Knowledge of your medical history
- Recognition of your rights and responsibilities as a patient

Although the primary responsibility and necessary knowledge for delivering safe care remains with your hospital and your doctor, you have a responsibility to follow instructions and to monitor your medical care. Your participation can have a major impact in preventing errors and infections.[7]

GOOD COMMUNICATION

Protecting your personal stake in safe care requires establishing good communication with all of your healthcare providers. This helps you to obtain complete information about your medical condition and participate in making decisions along the way. Several studies have shown that patients who are well informed about their health problems and satisfied with the care and communications from their healthcare providers experience a better treatment outcome than do those who are ill informed and dissatisfied with their care and communication.[8] I also know from a review of malpractice claims filed against doctors and hospitals that a lack of communication between the patient and his or her doctor is often the deciding factor in a patient's decision of whether to file a lawsuit.[9]

Ideally, your doctors and healthcare workers will offer explanations without being asked, and your hospital's staff will have been trained to encourage open communication with patients.[10] But don't count on it. Even if you're not accustomed to questioning doctors or other authority figures, this is the time to make an exception. When in doubt, ask! It could save your life.

Your Questions: What kinds of questions should you ask? As one example, just knowing the accurate name of your medical condition isn't enough. You need to ask what it means to have congestive heart failure, stage 3 breast cancer, a herniated disc, or any other medical problem.

Your Treatments: Are you sure you know exactly what treatment you'll receive in the hospital? If it's medication, what kind? What effects will it have on your body—both good benefits and bad risks? How will the treatment be administered? Especially if it's an antibiotic, ask why it's required and how long you will need it. Are there other drugs or treatments that would work just as well?

Feel Free to Ask . . .

Ideally, your doctors and healthcare workers will offer explanations without being asked.

But don't count on it. When in doubt, ask! It could save your life.

Your Surgery: If you're having surgery, you should be told what the surgeon will do. Remove an organ? Repair a heart valve? Replace a joint? Will you have a scar from an incision (a surgical cut through your skin) or will the surgery be done with instruments inserted through your mouth, anus, or another opening? Are there alternative treatments that wouldn't require surgery? What complications could occur and what would be done to correct them? What are your chances of having a total or partial recovery? How long will that take? What care will you require in the hospital, before and after surgery, and after you leave the hospital? Finally, what is your infection rate for my procedure?

Your Information: Many doctors and hospitals will provide printed fact sheets or video discs for you to take home, so you can review important information and gain a better understanding of the treatment you will receive. If you can't understand the information, ask your doctor to explain complicated medical jargon in simple words suitable for your education level and language abilities. If no one offers these materials or explanations to you, ask if any are available. If not, ask your local librarian for help researching the topic in print publications and online at reliable websites.

Your Costs: Also be sure to ask in advance how much your hospital care will cost, including fees for your hospital room, operating room (if required), tests, and medications, and for each of the doctors who may provide services during your stay. Are these costs covered by your medical insurance? If not, what assistance or payment plans are available to help you manage the hospital bills? Most insurance companies negotiate lower fees with hospitals and doctors, but patients without insurance who pay directly are often charged higher fees. If you ask, you may be able to negotiate lower fees for yourself.

No matter how sick you are, you have the right to know—and understand— what is being done to you, and why, and what it will cost. If you haven't been given the information you need, it's your responsibility to ask.

Doctors Can't Read Your Mind!

The U.S. Agency for Healthcare Research and Quality wants you to remember that doctors can't read your mind. In one of several humorous videos on their website (http://www.ahrq. gov/questions/video/restaurant15/), an assertive woman asks numerous questions to the waiter in a restaurant about how her meal will be prepared, if she can substitute the side item, and can she get the sauce on the side but hesitates to speak up at her doctor's office when her physician asks if she has any questions. If you're like that, perhaps you just don't know what to ask. Here are some suggested questions to start you off:

1. What is the test for?
2. How many times have you done this procedure?
3. When will I get the results?
4. Why do I need this treatment?
5. Are there any alternatives?
6. What are the possible complications?
7. Which hospital is best for my needs?
8. How do you spell the name of that drug?
9. Are there any side effects?

Check the Agency for Healthcare Research and Quality (AHRQ) website for more videos and more of their "Right Questions to Ask," or search YouTube for "AHRQ questions" for a number of short video clips on asking the right questions.

Q: I'm afraid that doctors and nurses will get angry if I ask too many questions. How can I be sure it's OK to ask?

A: I know it takes courage to ask questions and, especially, to voice complaints. I'm here to encourage you. In fact, in a study at a large hospital in Switzerland, over 75 percent of patients said they wouldn't feel comfortable asking nurses or doctors to wash their hands. But when a healthcare worker gave them a direct invitation to ask questions, almost 80 percent of patients said they would do so. Consider this as your direct invitation from me!

Q: Even when patients are given permission to ask questions, do many people actually do it?

A: In my work with hospitals in the United States and abroad, I was among the first infection control experts to study whether encouraging patients to ask questions could increase healthcare workers' hand-washing. I've found that 80 percent of Americans will ask questions and remind healthcare workers to wash their hands if they are given encouragement to do so.[11] Usually all it takes is simple training for healthcare workers to take the lead in empowering patients by providing simple instructions (as easy as giving the patient a brochure or inviting to ask questions). This fosters a productive patient–healthcare worker partnership where everybody wins. You get safer care, the hospital's costs in treating mistakes is reduced, and healthcare workers can focus on the jobs they like best—helping people!

Many hospitals conduct training programs for their doctors, nurses, and other staff members, encouraging them to communicate with patients. Doctors and nurses are busy people who are on call to respond to numerous patients' needs, so don't be offended if a healthcare worker seems rushed while speaking with you. Most medical professionals are dedicated, conscientious people who do care about their patients. So don't be afraid to ask questions.

Some hospital admissions offices provide a brochure for entering patients that explains the training program and gives patients "written permission" so they won't be afraid to ask questions. If your hospital doesn't provide these helpful guidelines, don't let that stop you. Be polite and non-confrontational, but do ask any important question that comes up.

If you don't have the courage to question doctors and nurses, consider appointing an advocate to help you. We talk about advocates next.

WHO SPEAKS FOR THE PATIENT?

If you're too weak or too upset to ask questions or to pay attention to the medical care you're receiving, you may need a health advocate.

Your advocate can be a family member, or close friend, or even a paid professional who can accompany you on visits to the doctor and during your hospital stay to help you get the information and care you need.

Your Advocate

The director of the AHRQ recommends that advocates should play an active role in your care, rather than serving as just "another set of ears and eyes" in your hospital room.[12] For example, health advocates can

- Help you make decisions about your medical care
- Ask questions or voice concerns to your doctor and other healthcare workers on your behalf, especially when you are incapacitated
- Keep written records of discussions with your doctors and a daily diary of tests, procedures, and incidents during your hospital stay
- Complete the paperwork requested by the hospital or your medical insurance company
- Monitor your medication regimen and help you follow treatment instructions
- Make certain that you are eating, drinking, urinating, and defecating regularly
- Ensure that you get your fair share of nursing care time and attention
- Alert doctors and nurses to changes in your symptoms and medical condition
- Report and document errors and care problems

That's just a start. When you're too ill to notice, your health advocate can be the one to remind healthcare workers to wash their hands. When you need a bedpan or attention to a problem and no one is answering your patient call button, your advocate can walk to the nursing station and ask for assistance. And much more.

Bring an Advocate

You can take a person with you to be your advocate. Be sure to choose someone who will be as reliable and caring as a dog would be. And tell your advocate to remind all your doctors, nurses, healthcare workers, and visitors to wash their hands before putting their hands on you.

Although many of these tasks are easy for anyone to do, this is not a job to be taken lightly. Being a health advocate requires a considerable commitment of time, the intelligence to understand medical information, careful attention to details, and a thorough knowledge of the patient's wishes, preferences, and beliefs. That's why it's best to choose someone who has known you well for many years. Set aside time before your hospitalization to discuss your care wishes with your advocate. That way you can be confident that the advocate will be guided by your preferences, rather than his or her own beliefs and values.

Your Living Will

One way to ensure that your advocate knows your wishes is with a living will. Do you have a living will and a healthcare proxy? Most hospitals now ask this question of every patient during the admissions process. A living will (in legal terms, an *advance directive*) is a signed legal document that indicates what kinds of treatment you would want, or not want, in the event you become unable to speak for yourself.[13] Usually this comes into play only in life or death situations. But even if you don't expect serious problems during your hospitalization, you may want to share your living will with your health advocate . . . just in case.

Your Proxy

A healthcare proxy is a related legal form by which you appoint a specific person (often referred to as your agent or your healthcare proxy) to make decisions on your behalf when you are incapacitated. Your agent can speak for you if there are questions about interpreting the wishes stated in your living will, so it's good to have both documents.[14] You could choose your agent as your advocate, but there's no requirement to do so.

An Advocate in the House

If you can't find anyone to be your advocate, you can appoint a nurse or doctor to fill this role. Choosing a healthcare professional is especially helpful if you and your family members have difficulty in understanding medical information. Your hospital personnel office may be able to recommend a staff member who does advocacy work as a paid or volunteer assignment.[15]

The following three questions can help you to understand the role of an advocate:[16]

Q: Do I need approval to bring an advocate with me into the hospital or a doctor's office?

A: You don't need approval to have someone with you in a doctor's office or examination room. Many doctors are accustomed to this. Hospital policies vary, so ask your doctor about it before you're admitted.

Q: What instructions should I give to my advocate?

A: Before your doctor's appointment or hospital admission, talk with your advocate about what you're worried about, what you think will be happening (for example, paperwork, medical tests, X-rays, etc.), and what help you want (such as taking notes, reminding you of questions you have, and asking questions for you).

Q: My surgery will be very minor, even though I have to stay in the hospital. If I'm conscious and alert, does my advocate still have the right to speak for me?

A: Most people wouldn't want an advocate to make requests or decisions for them if they're perfectly able to speak for themselves. Give your advocate instructions in advance about what you would, or would not, want him or her to do for you in each circumstance.

DON'T FORGET YOUR HISTORY!

If it's been 10 years or more since you were a hospital patient, you may be expecting regular visits from your personal physician during your hospitalization. Times have changed, and so has hospital care. Today, many hospitals rely on medical doctors called *hospitalists* to treat and monitor every patient. Because hospitalists usually spend most or all of the work day in the hospital, they're more available to care for you than your own doctor who is based outside the hospital.[17,18] With hospitalists on the job, your own doctor may not make many hospital visits to check on you.

Hospitalists receive extra training to specialize in the treatment of hospital patients, and studies have shown that reliance on hospitalists leads to "modest improvements" in the quality of hospital care, as well as cost savings.[19] But this may not be any comfort to you when you have to remind the hospitalist about aspects of your medical history and family situation that could affect your care—facts your personal physician knows first hand.

Get a Digital Copy of Your Medical History

That's why it's important for you to have an up-to-date medical history record in your possession. Many doctors' offices and hospitals have computerized their medical records and can give you a computer disc that contains all of your medical information. If that's not available, ask your doctor for a summary of important entries in your medical records and a list of your current medications. Be sure to include copies of recent tests, X-rays, and scans you've had so you won't waste time and money having them done again.

Use a Website

Are you planning to take a laptop with you to the hospital? Many websites on the Internet allow you to input your medical information and permanently save it online so it will be available to you or your healthcare team in an emergency. Some "patient-centered" web services also provide links to websites where you can get additional information and explanations about your medical conditions.[20]

One site that I have used for our family is www.accessmyrecords.com. Enter information from your own records and those your doctor gives you, and then create your own password. Only you will have access to your information unless you give it to someone, such as the advocate who will be with you in the hospital.

INFORMED CONSENT

At this point, you may be thinking you've done all that and you're well prepared and competent to face your hospital stay. Don't be so sure! Your biggest challenge is still to come: informed consent.

Each day we face the need to make informed decisions and provide consent. For example, the process of choosing a cellular telephone company or cable TV plan involves waiting in line, or on the phone, or scouring the Web to determine the best plan at the best price. The final step in that negotiation is a contract that explains (usually in such great detail that you practically need a lawyer to decipher it!) the conditions of the plan. Having reviewed all that information, you can make the decision to find another provider or confirm your consent to the current terms by signing the contract.

Rent a car? You'll have to sign a consent form. Your child wants to go on a field trip at school? You'll have to sign a consent form. Want to sign up to watch movies online? That's right; a signed consent form will be required. (Well, okay, actually you're "agreeing to the terms and conditions" of the software manufacturer, but for the sake of argument, it's pretty much a consent form.)

Too Much Trust

We use consent forms almost every day, and sometimes many times daily. So why do people have so much trouble applying the same skills and experience when it comes to consent forms for medical care? The answer is simply that we have placed too much trust in our healthcare providers, so we're willing to give them consent to treat us without our being fully informed. This unquestioning trust isn't related to a patient's age, level of education, or social background. In my opinion, it's the result of poor communication skills on the part of our doctors.

Informed consent is an agreement between you and your healthcare provider (the hospital and the doctors) for a proposed medical treatment, or a proposed invasive procedure, or a decision to have no treatment at the present time. It requires physicians to disclose the benefits, risks, and alternatives to the proposed treatment, procedure, or no treatment. It is the method by which fully informed, rational people can become involved in choices about their healthcare. It is a legal document in all 50 states.

Rights and Responsibilities

Did you know that it is the doctor's responsibility to engage patients in a dialogue that will encourage questions and learning? It's part of the Patient's Bill of Rights statutes that have been officially adopted by 23 states in the United States, and also independently adopted by a majority of hospitals throughout the country.[21]

73

Informed Consent Forms

Most hospital consent forms are long documents printed in tiny type, with many paragraphs written in hard-to-understand medical jargon. The first time most patients see one of these forms is when they're sitting the hospital admissions office before being taken to their hospital room. That's a big problem!

When you sit in that chair, you're already committed to being hospitalized, so it's psychologically difficult to change your mind at the last minute. And it's even more difficult to take enough time to read the small print, to try to understand what it means, and to decide whether you agree with everything in it.

Don't let that happen to you! Call your hospital and ask them to send you a copy of the consent form well before the day you're admitted. Take time to review it with your doctor. If you don't understand or agree with what's included, it's legal for you to cross out items you won't consent to.

Although provisions vary from state to state and hospital to hospital, the basic principle of informed consent is that you have the right, consistent with law, to "receive all the information that you need to give informed consent for any proposed procedure or treatment. This information shall include the possible risks and benefits of the procedure or treatment."

Your Role

As patients, we can no longer accept our doctors' words under the umbrella of "Trust me, I know what's best for you." It's your legal right to obtain all the relevant information you need before signing on the dotted line of a medical consent form. But it's also your personal responsibility to request this information and to work with your healthcare team to follow their recommendations and take good care of yourself.

THIS EXPERT FAILED THE TEST

I have been involved in healthcare for more than 30 years. I'm definitely familiar with the process of informed consent. So, when my husband needed heart bypass surgery after a heart attack, (a common procedure, but potentially difficult and even life-threatening), I felt confident that I could be an excellent advocate for him by asking all the important questions that concerned me.

"Fast Track"

Of course, as an infection preventionist, I asked about the hospital's infection rates and recent infection outbreaks. When I learned that five patients in the cardiac unit had infections, I insisted my husband be placed in a separate room, away from the infected patients, which meant that he would stay only a short time in the critical care area. Very sick patients often remain there, so there's a high risk of other patients catching an infection. I wanted to protect my husband.

I felt good about my skills as an advocate. I was given the information I needed, and all of my requests were granted, so my husband signed the consent form agreeing to bypass surgery. Everything went well!

A Surprise

So why am I telling this story? Because a year later, when we were living in England, we had a shocking surprise. When my husband needed a checkup, he was examined by a well-respected cardiologist in the hospital at which I was a visiting researcher. After looking at my husband's medical records and imaging scans, the cardiologist very matter-of-factly asked, "Why did you have a bypass operation? You clearly had only peripheral disease. This certainly would not warrant bypass surgery."

We were dumbfounded. It might be argued that bypass surgery was the right operation for my husband at that time or that this new cardiologist's opinion reflected the British system of healthcare. But the critical issue was that we never asked the really important questions: "Is this surgery necessary?" and "Are there any alternatives?"

Ask the Questions

I'm a healthcare professional; why didn't I think to ask those questions? Because there never seemed to be the opportunity to do so. We were continually told how lucky my husband was to have a second chance at life, thanks to bypass surgery. We were reminded that many patients never survive a heart attack, but he was the lucky one, he was getting a second chance. This type of dialogue did not open a channel for communication. If we had voiced any questions to the contrary, we might have been seen as ungrateful.

Even as educated professionals, it never crossed our minds that the people who would be performing this surgery were the same ones who were providing information to reassure us that surgery was the right choice. We were never given all the facts, alternatives, and the opportunity for an unbiased provider–patient dialogue before we signed the consent form for my husband to undergo surgery. We asked many questions but we didn't think to get a second or third opinion from other top cardiologists. But when you are frightened and thinking only about surviving, the first offer of hope is often the one you believe is best. Even 14 years later, both my husband and I still question that decision.

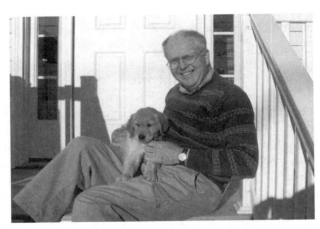

Husband Jack and his Buddy.

What did we learn from that situation? After our return to the United States, the first thing we did was to find a new cardiologist. This time, we interviewed each candidate before selecting the specialist who would treat my husband. If a cardiologist described his care plan for my husband and implied, "This is how I treat all of my patients, and it's not up for discussion," that doctor was immediately "fired before hired."

Schedule a Visit

We did find a wonderful cardiologist and for 13 years he was a resource and friend. Unfortunately, in 2010, this wonderful cardiologist died and we learned very quickly an important fact: Don't think all doctors in a practice are the same and will fill your needs. You need to meet with each doctor before you transfer your care. My husband's approach was to have a scheduled office visit with his former cardiologist's partner; in fact, he had at least three visits and then realized this was not a good fit.

With his reliable records in hand, we began another search. After doing some research and with my recommendation, we saw another cardiologist. We provided this cardiologist with records prior to the visit. However, after the first visit, we once again knew this was not a good fit. No communication, no efforts to discuss alternatives, and most disturbing was a feeling of it being a virtual visit. He asked questions "toward" my husband, while entering every word into his laptop, creating a new electronic medical record. No need for Jack to be at the visit; we could have done this over the phone or via a computer questionnaire.

A Good Fit ... or Not

On our third try, we thought we found a good fit. We used every form of empowerment. We called the medical director of the hospital and asked for a recommendation. We were given two names and I emailed the first one, detailing our needs and the fact that he would receive all records, which we expected him to review before our visit. If this could not be done, we would not make an appointment. I also made sure that I copied the email to the medical director, his superior. Even though I'm a health professional, anyone including you or your advocate can make these calls and emails to inquire about a new specialist. Amazingly, it worked! I received an email a week before the visit, saying he reviewed all records and had a plan. All went well on our first visit. However, we quickly discovered when we called the office that this was a private practice with a name very similar to a hospital, but had no affiliation with the hospital. The hospital's medical director had given us an off-site reference without specifying they had no relationship with the hospital itself. It was clearly a profit practice in which there were at least a dozen cardiologists, many nurses, assistants, etc., and they offered—or should I say tried to "sell"—every high-tech procedure and advised that after our first appointment, our contact would be a nurse. In the health services sector, there are many off-site offices and services that are legitimately affiliated with a healthcare system, and the doctors are often paid by the hospital. Then there are others that have practices near a hospital, have admitting privileges but operate financially as independent corporations and for profits. Many perform well and must follow the same compliance rules as the big health systems but we have found that their care plan involves more testing than necessary. So, I am sad to report that we are still looking. Is it difficult to do this? Yes! And do I feel like I am seen as an aggressive wife? Of course I do. But my goals were a good outcome for my husband and living up to my role as an advocate. However, I am pleased to report that after our second failed attempt, my husband has become an excellent advocate for himself and I know will be there for me.

The Other Side of the Knife

I believe that the major reason for the superior, 13-year relationship we had with his former cardiologist is the fact that, like my husband, he also had a heart attack at a young age and underwent bypass surgery. He's learned the value of communication. As he often told his patients, he's been "on the other side of the knife."

YOUR "TOP SIX" LIST

I'm sure that many of you have signed an informed consent form, with complete faith in your doctor and in the information you received. Even under adverse circumstances, the outcome was probably good. That's what we all hope for. Still, you can't expect that everything will always turn out well. Healthcare-associated infections will always occur, as will unintentional errors, and surgeries that don't bring relief. That doesn't mean healthcare workers were negligent; it's just that the world is an imperfect place.

However, healthcare is constantly changing and not always for the better. We are faced with shortages of doctors, nurses, and other healthcare professionals, as well as constantly increasing medical costs. The harsh reality is that patients in the United States receive optimal medical care only 50 percent of the time.[5]

That means you can no longer afford the luxury of signing an informed consent document just because you're asked to, or it's a requirement, or you don't want to seem uncooperative. I've been there, done that, and regretted it. Now I know to ask better questions and insist on unbiased answers before putting my signature on the dotted line. Here's what you need to ask:

The Six Things You *Must Know* Before Signing an Informed Consent Form[22]

1. The patient's diagnosis (if known)
2. The type and purpose of the proposed treatment or procedure
3. The risks and benefits of not receiving the treatment or undergoing the procedure
4. The risks and the benefits of undergoing the treatment or procedure
5. The alternatives to treatment (regardless of costs or insurance coverage)
6. The risks and benefits of these alternatives to the suggested treatment or procedure

---

The information you receive must be in a language that you understand. If it isn't, ask for a better explanation or a translation. Be sure that you are satisfied with the answers to those six items. If an answer isn't satisfactory to you—for example, if you were told that there are no alternatives except for the treatment suggested by the hospital—write that on the form before you sign it. The informed consent form is a legal document that hospitals and healthcare providers can, and often will, use against you if anything goes wrong. If you sign the form, hospital personnel can say that you knew the risks before treatment and that you gave your consent anyway. So make sure the answers to your six questions satisfy all of your concerns.

Except in an emergency situation, hospitals and healthcare providers will not treat you until you give them permission to do so—that is, until you have provided informed consent. Your signature on an informed consent form means that you have discussed each of the "Six Things You *Must Know* Before Signing an Informed Consent Form."

If you're not completely satisfied with what you've been told, don't let anyone pressure you into signing.

In most hospitals, you will be asked to sign a "blanket form," which applies to all the treatments you may undergo while you are receiving hospital care. That means you're giving the hospital staff and physicians permission to do anything they feel is necessary during your stay. I recommend asking for a "single-treatment form," which applies to only the one treatment or procedure you are currently undergoing, such as a knee replacement or a heart operation. In fact, courts have ruled that blanket forms are too unclear. You should give permission only for what you feel is medically necessary, correct, and good for you.

Q: Can I make changes to the informed consent document before I sign it?

A: Yes. You can make changes to, and write in questions about, the terms of the consent form. For example, you might not know it, but interns and residents frequently perform surgery.

The catch phrase in medical school is, "See one, do one, teach one." The attending surgeon must be present during a surgical procedure (or at least, that's what the law says), but the one who actually performs the surgery may be an intern or a resident. That's how students learn surgical technique. That might be your surgery.

So, if you're having a hip replacement and you don't want anyone but your own surgeon to perform that procedure, you can add a line to your consent form stating that no intern or resident is to perform your surgery. Bear in mind that the hospital or doctor won't necessarily like this, but you have the right to do it nevertheless. If you need assistance in making your wishes known, insist on speaking to a patient representative or advocate.

Most hospitals have such personnel whose sole job is to resolve problems. Remember: It's your right.

Q: Can a hospital refuse to admit me if I don't sign a consent form? Do I lose my legal rights when I sign a blanket form?

A: In this situation, hospitals will often try to make you sign a general release form stating that you assume responsibility if something goes wrong with your treatment. However, U.S. courts have said that those releases aren't legal because they are often signed under pressure. For example, you are in pain and need surgery, but the hospital will not schedule the necessary procedure until you have signed a general release form. Clearly, you are not in a position to bargain in that situation.

The courts have also specified that you should be given adequate time to discuss and ask questions about informed consent. Therefore, documents that you signed under distress are not considered binding. Always remember:

- Do not sign a consent form unless you or your advocate has a clear understanding of its content and has had sufficient time to discuss the six things that you *must know* before providing informed consent.
- If you are not satisfied, ask to speak to the patient representative or advocate.
- If this is not an emergency situation, get a second opinion.

Finally, if you have a complaint about a hospital or you are concerned about the quality of care you have received, contact the Joint Commission, which sets standards for hospitals and also enforces patients' rights. You can email the Joint Commission at compliant@jointcommission.org, send them a fax at (630) 792-5636, or mail your complaint to:

Office of Quality Monitoring
The Joint Commission
One Renaissance Blvd.
Oakbrook Terrace, IL 60181

Summarize the issue in two pages or less and include the name and full address of the hospital in question. For more information, call the Joint Commission's toll free number, (800) 994-6610, available weekdays, 8:30 a.m. to 5 p.m., Central Time.

An investigation that might include an unannounced visit to the healthcare facility will be conducted, but your information will remain confidential.

Four Things You Must Know About Informed Consent

1. Never sign a blank form. Informed consent documents should be specific to your treatment or procedure.
2. You can make changes to consent documents.
3. You do not lose your legal rights by signing a form.
4. If your hospital or doctor is not willing to discuss the six things that you *must know* before signing an informed consent form, then find another hospital and doctor.

MEET KERRY O'CONNELL, AN INFORMED AND EMPOWERED PATIENT

The goal of this chapter was to help you become an empowered patient. That's why I want you to know about Kerry O'Connell, a man who is that and much more. Here is his story and the courageous battle he won. Yes, I say won, because he took his experience with a healthcare-associated infection to help get laws passed in his state to protect other patients.

In Kerry's Own Words

October 30, 2004 was a glorious fall Saturday high in the Colorado foothills. I was up on a ladder painting away with only one more side of the house to finish. As I climbed down 17 feet to move the decrepit ladder over, I noticed that its broken legs were digging into my new asphalt driveway. It was then that I embarked on the stupidest act of my entire life: I placed some cardboard under the legs.

After climbing back up, I made two passes with the spray gun then found myself lying face first on the asphalt unable to breathe. After an eternity of oxygen starvation, I caught a breath and tried to push myself up to my knees. My left arm crushed under the weight of my body . . . I yelled for help and luckily, Anne and the kids had not left for Halloween parties at the malls. (She) drove my battered hyperventilating body a mile to the Conifer Medical Center.

Call in the Clowns

It took Doctor No. 1 and three nurses in Halloween clown costumes every bit of strength they had to pull my arm apart so the dislocated elbow would slide back into place. Once reduced, the arm really did not feel bad at all . . . .

(*Two days later*) on Monday morning, I went the big ortho clinic in Golden, Colorado, that the initial doctor (No. 1) had recommended. They . . . said I needed to see their hand specialist . . . (Doctor No. 2), who said my radial head (a bone near the elbow) was cracked and might need to be cut off and a titanium implant installed. Didn't sound too bad . . . . I woke up (after surgery) . . . with tubes everywhere, a metal fixator contraption on my arm, and massive pain throughout my arm and head.

(When) Doctor No. 2 came in looking extremely ill, I asked him how it went. He said "OK." I told him it looked like they put the maximum amount of hardware on me (and) he said, "Yeah, we had to." Then, he left without another word. The next morning I discovered my wrist and fingers were totally limp. Four and a half months later, my third doctor would

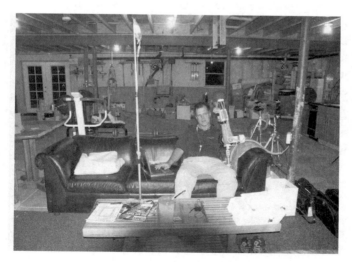

This is how Kerry lived for 18 months after his methicillin-resistant *Staphylococcus aureus* (MRSA) infection.

discover that the bone drill had pureed 4 inches of my radial nerve into mush.

(Next came) surgery number two in April, . . . a futile attempt to splice 3 parallel pieces of the spaghetti size sural nerve from my left calf into the 4-inch void in my radial nerve. We knew it had less than a 5 percent chance of working (and it didn't) . . . .

Infection and More Surgery

Somehow my faith in doctors was still stronger than my faith in God, and (in August) I went full steam ahead . . . for surgery number 3, elbow capsulectomy, to restore range of motion in my very stiff elbow . . . (It) resulted in a very serious MRSA infection. It took two months, four more surgeries, and many gallons of vancomycin to kill the bacteria in my arm. Doctor No. 3 had to take out my titanium implant, but at least I still had my stiff arm and limp hand.

By December, we were confident that the MRSA was gone and the nerve graft was not going to work. (With great determination and great terror, I asked Doctor No. 3 to perform tendon transfer surgery.) On December 9th, (as) I lay in the pre-op center . . . the physician's assistant and Doctor No. 3 could not quite remember which tendons we had agreed to move. By this point, I had become highly informed (so) I handed them my spreadsheet, pointed excitedly (to the right tendons), and prayed.

God had finally tested me enough and allowed this surgery to work. I spent another 4 months in physical therapy and wound up with a 70-percent elbow and a 60-percent hand, which works pretty well considering that 10 of the 40 muscles in my arm will never work again.

What Kerry Learned

I had drilled enough things in my life to fully comprehend how bone drills could slip and destroy nerves. Similarly, I had fought enough battles with mold in buildings to understand how difficult it is to control bacteria. Yet what completely astounded me was the medical community's reaction when things go wrong. Taking responsibility is out of the question. The best they could muster was to weakly blame the fixator manufacturer and hospital staff while sending me truly outrageous bills.

It appears that this profession, which was founded on love, has been totally consumed by fear and greed. In response, I started writing letters, giving speeches, and supporting legislation to try to remind physicians how to love their patients when things go wrong.

Here's One of the Letters Kerry Wrote to Legislators

April 14, 2008

Since surviving a tough battle with MRSA in the fall of 2005, about a third of my waking thoughts are consumed with the question of how do you win the war with the invisible enemy called bacteria . . . The experts all agree that there are no easy answers, no miracle cures, and no silver bullets. I helped to pass the infection reporting law in Colorado, but have come to believe that we cannot write laws that are detailed enough, flexible enough, or tough enough to win this war.

In the past two decades, we have witnessed the corporate takeover of healthcare. Interestingly, corporations are very much like bacteria. Both exist for the sole purpose of growth and survival. The means for corporate survival has always been and will always be profitability . . . Consider the two things that you will never hear come out of a healthcare CEO's mouth:

1. We made too much money this year!
2. We lost money this year but that is acceptable because we didn't harm any patients!

The plan to win the war is simple. Make infection prevention highly profitable. Currently, this nation spends about $4 billion dollars a year treating 2 million infections, which at 7 percent profit equates to about $280 million dollars a year in healthcare profits. Most experts would agree that if we spent that same $4 billion a year on prevention measures, infections would be nearly extinct. The problem is that no insurance company or centers for Medicare and Medicaid would pay for $4 billion *in prevention measures, because the resulting $8 billion dollar swing from revenue to overhead would bankrupt a lot of providers.*

My solution is [that we should] quit paying $2,000 per patient to treat the unlucky souls that get infected and instead give the providers a $25 bonus for every patient they don't infect. They then get the $5 billion in revenue that is now distributed to the providers with the best rates, instead of going to the facilities with the worst rates. Infections will become extremely hazardous to the bottom line. Corporate healthcare, like bacteria, will quickly adapt, morph, and change into mean, clean, bacteria-killing machines.

The providers that I have proposed this to have an interesting response: "But would we have to share the bonus with the doctors?" Again the profit-centered culture. The right answer is, "Yes, of course," as doctors (especially surgeons) are integral to stopping infections.

No one will argue that hospitals are grossly understaffed in infection control, that screening takes money, and that isolation wings cost big money. Give them the funds to fight the war effectively and quit rewarding them for failures!

Sincerely,

Kerry O'Connell

BRING ON CONSUMER POWER!

As you can see in the picture of Kerry at home, he had a long, difficult battle with his infection. Kerry gets an A-plus for his empowerment, his determined efforts to recover, and for successfully being able to change laws in Colorado. Unfortunately, we are now seeing that laws aren't the full answer. Indeed, Medicaid is beginning to deny payments to hospitals for certain healthcare-associated infections, but I'm not sure the idea of self-reporting of errors is the best way to reward healthcare facilities that do a good job.

It's often said that the next big change in healthcare will be driven by consumers. Kerry is a consumer who proves that point. It takes a strong will like Kerry's to change things. Maybe you will be the next person who makes that happen!

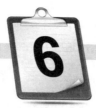

Infection Protection When You
Need a Urinary Catheter

Now that you've learned about the many actions you can take to prevent infections, are you ready to tackle the kinds of infections you might face as a hospital patient? Because urinary infections are the most common healthcare-associated infections, I'll start with them and then go on to prevention of other infections that affect many hospital patients. Here's the agenda for the next few chapters:

1. Urinary tract infections (UTIs) associated with urinary catheters
2. Respiratory infections and ventilator-associated pneumonia (VAP)
3. Surgical site infections (SSIs)
4. Bloodstream infections associated with venous catheters (BSI)

INTERVENTIONAL PATIENT HYGIENE

Because the healthcare-associated infection types listed above are so common, I co-developed with other health researchers a model for patient hygiene that assigns hygiene treatment for each common infection.[1] Sounds simple, and is simple to follow, but as you have read already, healthcare workers for various reasons will not, cannot, or forget to follow simple hygiene procedures.

Start with the middle of the diagram on the next page which represents the patient—you! Then the next layer that surrounds (and protects) the patient are the three types of hygiene interventions you and your

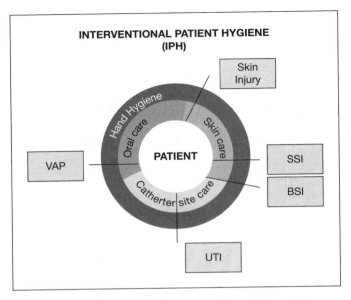

Components and outcomes of the IPH model.

healthcare team must practice: oral care, skin care, and catheter site care. In other words, proper oral hygiene, skin bathing (remember those chlorhexidine wipes!) and keeping clean the area of your body at and around the catheter insertion point, are crucial to protecting that patient at the center of the model.

The outer circle that surrounds the three types of patient hygiene is the most frequently performed hygiene procedure I have discussed time and again: hand hygiene! Healthcare workers must wash or sanitize their hands before performing any other hygiene treatment such as teeth cleaning, skin cleaning, or cleaning at the catheter site. If a healthcare worker does any of these procedures with unclean hands, then they are simply passing hand bacteria and viruses onto your newly cleaned skin, mouth, or catheter site.

Note the infections (VAP, BSI, UTI, SSI, and skin injury) in the boxes surrounding the circles. These are the infections that are kept away from the patient thanks to the protecting hygiene interventions noted in the shaded circle segments around the patient. For example, UTI (urinary tract infections) are kept away from the patient by performing proper catheter site care and hand hygiene. Surgical site infections (SSI) are kept away from the patient by proper skin care and hand hygiene. Blood stream infections

(BSI) are kept away from the patient by performing proper skin care AND catheter site care, along with hand hygiene.

If healthcare workers practiced these simple hygiene interventions (oral, skin, and catheter site), you, the patient, will have a better chance of avoiding infections. Don't forget, you can be a part of that "protecting team" by reminding your healthcare workers to wash or sanitize their hands, and by ensuring your bathing routine is performed daily.

CAN'T GO WITH THE FLOW

OK, here's your first infection challenge. Whether you call it urinating, emptying your bladder, or voiding, it's something most people do several times a day without giving it much thought. But for people who are hospitalized, urinating may involve effort, discomfort, and sometimes the need for a urinary catheter.

What causes these problems? First, imagine trying to urinate while sitting on a hospital bedpan, as some hospital patients must do. If you've ever done it, you know how strange and uncomfortable it can be. Many people can't get urine to flow in that position. Next, your ability to urinate can be affected if you've had surgery or have a medical problem affecting your bladder, prostate or penis (in men), uterus or vagina (in women), or any organ in the area near your pelvic region. That's why you may notice thin tubing draining your urine into a plastic bag when you wake up after surgery.

WHAT'S HAPPENING DOWN THERE?

You can easily see the catheter tube leading outside of your body, but you may not understand where it's located inside your body and what it's doing there.[2] Your kidneys are located over the bladder. That's where urine is formed. The kidneys filter waste and water out of your bloodstream. The urine then flows down from each kidney via thin tube-like structures called ureters (one on each side) and ends up in the balloon-shaped bladder.

The bladder stretches as it fills with urine. If everything is working right, urine won't continually drip out into the urethra tube below, thanks to a sphincter muscle that holds the bladder closed. But when the bladder is full, it's time for the nerves in the bladder wall to send signals through the spinal cord to the brain and back to the bladder. That starts contractions and relaxes the sphincter muscle, so urine can flow down the urethra and out of the body.

Uh, oh! What if you're not near a toilet or a bedpan? Fortunately, there's another sphincter muscle at the end of the urethra that you can control yourself to hold the urine in. You've probably done this many times.

WHEN THINGS GO WRONG

That's how urination works when there are no medical problems. But here's what can go wrong:

- In men, if the prostate gland just under the bladder gets too large, it presses on the urethra and can block urine flow.
- In men and women, blockages in the urethra can occur from tumors, infections, scar tissue, and other causes.
- Spinal cord injuries, strokes, tumors, diabetes, infections, and other conditions can affect the nerves that control the bladder. This may prevent transmission of signals to empty the bladder.
- Some medications, particularly cold and allergy drugs containing ephedrine, can cause difficulty in urinating so the bladder becomes painfully overfull and doesn't empty. That's called urinary retention.

When you're in the hospital, other problems may arise. For example, if you have urologic surgery or operations on nearby organs in the lower abdominal area (the uterus, for example, during a cesarean section), you're likely to develop urinary retention. After-effects of anesthesia also increase your retention risks, and so does being immobile in a hospital bed.

IN'S AND OUT'S OF CATHETER USE

With so many possible problems that can interfere with urination, you may not be surprised to learn that as many as one out of every four hospitalized patients in the United States winds up with a urinary catheter during a hospital stay.[3]

The most common type is a *Foley catheter*, also called an indwelling urinary catheter. It consists of a long, soft plastic or rubber tube that is inserted into the urinary opening (at the tip of the penis in men and just under the clitoris in women). The tube is then passed up through the urethra and into the bladder. Next, a tiny balloon at the top of the tube is inflated with sterile water through a second tube to hold the catheter in place. When it's time to remove the catheter, the balloon is deflated and the tube is gently pulled out.[4]

The bottom of the catheter tube is connected to a drainage bag, which collects the urine that flows down the tube. Because of gravity, the bag must be kept below the level of the bladder, to prevent urine from flowing back up.[4]

Q: Are there other types of catheters?

A: Several types of urinary catheters are available:

- Intermittent (short-term) catheters are used for quick drainage of urine. Because the catheter doesn't have to stay in place, there's no balloon at the top.
- People who have a blockage in the urethra may need a suprapubic catheter, which is inserted directly into the bladder through a small hole that's made in the lower abdomen.
- Another type called a condom catheter, used mostly for men who are permanently incontinent (can't control urine flow), doesn't involve a tube inserted through the penis. Instead, a condom-like covering with a tube attached is placed over the penis. Urine flows down through the tube into a drainage bag. This type of catheter is easy to change and poses less risk of causing an infection.[4]

Other types of catheters are used to deliver medications into the bloodstream (venous catheters), monitor heart function (cardiac catheters), and drain fluids from the abdomen or chest. We'll talk more about these in the following chapters.

Q: Does it hurt to have a urinary catheter?

A: Urinary catheters come in different diameters—choosing the best size for each person helps to prevent discomfort. Before it's inserted, the catheter tube is coated with lubricant to help it pass easily, but most people still feel discomfort during insertion. Men especially often feel pain as the catheter passes through the prostate area. A topical anesthetic applied to the insertion area may be used to decrease any pain for both men and women. However, once the catheter is properly inserted, it should cause only minor discomfort.[5] If the catheter becomes painful, it needs to be replaced immediately.[4]

Catheters and Pain

When a urinary catheter is inserted properly, it should cause only slight discomfort.

Tell your doctor or nurse if it becomes painful. That means the catheter needs to be replaced immediately.

Q: Are there possible complications from having a catheter?

A: Some people develop allergic reactions to the latex used in catheter tubing and may need to switch to silicone tubing. Other possible complications include stones forming in the bladder, blood in the urine (hematuria), injury to the urethra, and, with long-term indwelling catheters, kidney damage. We also know that urinary catheters used in people older than 70 years are associated with an increased risk of death.[6] But the most common complication of all is infection in the urinary tract or kidneys.[4]

HOW CATHETERS CAUSE URINARY TRACT INFECTIONS

Each year, about 2.5 million hospitalized patients in the United States develop healthcare-associated infections. One million of these infections (30 percent) are UTIs, the majority of which are related to the use of urinary catheters. Any device that's inserted into a part of the body is an open highway for germs to move right in. That's the major reason why catheter-related infections are so common.[7]

Q: What is the urinary tract?

A: The kidneys, ureters, bladder, and urethra are part of the urinary tract.

Q: Do all patients who have a urinary catheter get an infection?

A: No, but we do know that for each day you have a catheter in place, you have a 3-7 percent chance of bacteria getting into your urine. This is called *bacteriuria*. Do the math: If your catheter is in place for 10 days, you'll have a 30-70 percent chance of getting bacteriuria.[7]

Q: Is bacteriuria the same as infection?

A: No, but if the bacteria continue to multiply and start causing symptoms, such as pain during urination, then you have developed an infection. From 10 to 25 percent of people who get bacteriuria do develop UTIs. In addition, approximately 3 percent of people who have bacteriuria develop *bacteremia*, a potentially fatal condition in which bacteria growing in the urine get into the bloodstream, where they can travel throughout the body. Because of possible bacteremia, people who develop bacteriuria can have a three-fold increased risk of dying.[8]

Q: Are some catheters better than others in preventing bacteriuria?

A: Catheters that are coated with silver alloy have been shown to decrease bacteriuria. This is probably because silver acts like an antimicrobial agent—it kills bacteria. Because silver alloy catheters are more expensive than standard ones, some hospitals use them only for intensive care patients.

Q: "More expensive" shouldn't matter. Aren't hospitals responsible for doing everything possible to prevent infections?

A: Before January 2008, most hospitals and doctors worked on the premise that catheter-related infections were not always preventable and therefore not a top priority in terms of trying to decrease their numbers. In fact, some hospitals viewed them as a way to generate money from additional treatments and longer hospital stays.

That changed as of October 2008, when Medicare created guidelines for what they categorized as preventable hospital conditions. UTIs fit those guidelines and so do other healthcare-associated infections. This means that hospitals can no longer be reimbursed for any additional costs of treating UTIs that Medicare and Medicaid patients acquire in the hospital if those infections are considered preventable. Hospitals and healthcare workers always work to prevent infections in all of their patients, but now they have an even greater incentive.[9]

Good News!

Hospitals really don't want you to develop a UTI.

There's a big incentive for preventing it, because Medicare and Medicaid will no longer reimburse the hospital for the added costs of treating hospital-associated UTIs.

HOW YOU CAN HELP

The Medicare guidelines are good news for every patient, because healthcare workers work to reduce infection in everyone, not just those on Medicare/Medicaid. In addition, hospital physicians and administrators in the United States are fully informed about other infection control guidelines issued by the World Health Organization[10] and the U.S. Centers for Disease Control and Prevention and its associated professional infection control organizations.[6,7] However, a recent survey of several hundred hospitals in the United States showed that the majority of hospitals weren't using even basic, proven practices to prevent hospital-associated UTIs.[11] That means it's important for you to play a part in making sure you don't get an infection when you're a patient yourself or when you're acting as an advocate, helping to protect another person.

The Centers for Disease Control supports and encourages this patient involvement. They've even issued patient guides on many kinds of health-care-associated infections to help people know how to take action.[12] Use this link to view the Centers for Disease Control and Prevention's Frequently Asked Questions (FAQs) About Catheter-Associated Urinary Tract Infection: http://www.cdc.gov/HAI/ca_uti/cauti_faqs.html.

Here's my professional FAQ advice that I give to people who may need a urinary catheter while they're hospitalized:

Q: What can a patient or advocate do to prevent a healthcare-associated UTI?

A: The first and most effective way is to avoid having a urinary catheter whenever possible. Even in critical care patients, use of a urinary catheter is often unjustified. But if you must have one, the catheter should remain in place for the shortest possible time. The longer a urinary catheter stays in, the greater the risk of infection.[13]

It's hard to believe, but studies show, that more than 50 percent of hospitals do not monitor the length of time catheters remain in place after they are inserted.[11] An even greater concern in one study is that over 50 percent of healthcare workers failed to specify the reason why each patient needed a catheter or failed to write down the exact date each patient's urinary catheter was first inserted.[14]

Some hospitals are responding to this problem with the simple practice of putting a reminder on patients' charts to alert healthcare workers when a urinary catheter is in use and to ask for a specific "stop" date when the catheter would be removed. Hospitals using this approach were able to decrease the duration of catheter usage by 37 percent and, in fact, decreased infections by 52 percent.[13]

Q: How can I know if a urinary catheter is really necessary?

A: If you can't empty your bladder, you need a catheter, but that doesn't mean you need it for a long time. Even if you can urinate normally, your doctor may order a catheter when your urine output needs to be monitored. Because the urine flows into a bag, it's easy to measure. Although catheters should be removed as soon as possible, orders for urine monitoring often aren't reviewed and canceled. As a result, each extra day you continue with the catheter means an additional 3–7 percent chance of getting bacteriuria.[7] You can help to prevent an infection by asking the doctor every day whether you still need the catheter and for what reason.

Q: How can I know when a urinary catheter isn't necessary?

A: Urinary catheters should not be used to obtain a urine specimen if a patient can void normally and should never be used as a substitute for nursing care. Healthcare workers often decide to keep patients catheterized when a shortage of staff members makes it more convenient to have patients void that way, rather than having to help them or having to change soiled bed linens. This is not good medical practice. Don't let it happen to you or anyone else!

Q: What should I watch for when my catheter is inserted or replaced?

A: It's important to keep the catheter clean and free from germs that cause infections. The biggest chance for bacteria to get into the catheter is when it's inserted. That's why inserting or replacing a catheter should be done only by properly trained people using sterile or "clean" technique.

When your catheter is being cleaned or replaced, make sure your nurse starts by washing his or her hands with soap and water or by using an alcohol-based sanitizer and then puts on fresh sterile gloves. Next, the nurse should clean your skin in the area where the catheter will be inserted before opening a sterile pack to remove a fresh catheter for insertion.

Watch every step carefully! For example, it sometimes happens that doctors and nurses will put sterile gloves on without first cleaning their hands or will remove a clean catheter from a sterile pack only to place it on a dirty tray. If you see something, say something!

Q: Are any precautions needed when the urine bag is emptied?

A: When urine must be taken from the bag or the bag needs to be emptied, the healthcare worker must clean his or her hands rather than just putting on gloves. When emptying the catheter or removing a urine sample, the catheter shouldn't be disconnected from the drain tube; this prevents bacteria from getting into the catheter tube. Also be sure that the drainage spout doesn't touch anything that could be dirty.

After emptying, the urine bag must be returned to a secure place below the patient, so that there is always a downward flow. If the bag is placed on top of your bed or on top of you in the bed, there is a chance of bacteria flowing upward into your body. But don't put it on the dirty floor! Check to see that there are no twists or kinks in the tubing. If the catheter stops draining urine into the bag, report it so the problem can be corrected.

DID YOU GET AN INFECTION?

Sometimes even careful hygiene isn't enough to prevent a catheter-related UTI. But when you're in the hospital recovering from illness or an operation and feeling generally uncomfortable, you may not even realize that you've developed an infection. Here's what you should look for:

- Redness or swelling around the area of the catheter. That can also be a sign that your catheter needs to be cleaned or changed.
- Burning or pain in your lower abdomen (below your stomach)
- Blood, stones, or sediment in your urine
- Fever or chills
- The catheter drains very little urine, even though you're drinking enough fluids

Don't wait to report a problem! While you're waiting, the infection keeps spreading. Of course, some of these symptoms could be caused by other problems, so check with a doctor or nurse to know for sure. If an infection is suspected, a sample of your urine will be sent to the laboratory to check for bacteria and identify which kinds of bacteria are present.

As this suggests, you can expect to be treated with antibiotics for any catheter-associated UTI. Not just any antibiotic will do. As you'll remember from reading about methicillin-resistant *Staphylococcus aureus* (MRSA), many strains of bacteria have become resistant to standard antibiotics. Accredited hospitals are required to keep records of which antibiotics have not been effective in treating recent bacterial infections in your geographic location. Be sure to ask if your doctor has checked these records to select the most effective antibiotic against the bacteria you're fighting. This is extremely important—it could save your life![15]

ONE MORE THING

Do all these instructions seem like too much to remember and too much to worry about? I've worked with hundreds of patients in hospitals all across the country, and I can assure you that it's not hard to protect yourself from infections. I know you CAN do it! In fact, there's just one basic thing you have to remember:

> *If you don't see healthcare workers wash or sanitize their hands before approaching your bedside, always ask them to do so.*

Actually, there *is* one more thing:

> *Always wash or sanitize your own hands frequently to keep them clean while you're in the hospital.*

If you remember these two simple things, you've already done most of the work. I told you it was easy.

To remind you of other infection-preventing strategies, here's a checklist you can take to the hospital in case you need a urinary catheter.

Checklist for Catheter-Associated UTI

- ❑ Remember to ask: *Do I need the urinary catheter?*
- ❑ Also ask: *How long will I need the catheter?*
- ❑ Remind yourself or your advocate to ask the doctor each day whether you still need the catheter and, if so, the reason you still need it.
- ❑ During catheter insertion, be sure the doctor or nurse starts with handwashing and is careful to keep the catheter sterile, within the sterile area, and not opened and placed down on your tray table.

- ❑ Keep the urine bag below you at all times.
- ❑ Remember the question: *Did you wash or sanitize your hands?*

WHAT WOULD YOU DO?

Now that you know the facts about catheter-associated UTIs, would you feel empowered to help yourself or a loved one who needs a urinary catheter during her hospital stay? Put on your own Sherlock Holmes, hat and read through this story about Julie Rich, told by her daughter. Would you have done anything different than what her daughter did?

Julie Rich's Story

My mother is 65 and she has always been very healthy. That is, until she went in for what was supposed to be simple, routine, day surgery.

Whenever Mother did heavy housework or lifted things, she kept wetting her pants. She didn't like wearing urine pads, so the doctor told her to have something called a sling put in to hold her bladder up. He arranged a morning appointment for her at our hospital's outpatient wing to have the sling surgery done.

When the surgery was finished, they sent her home wearing a catheter, but it didn't seem to be draining the urine out right. So after the weekend, we took Mother back to the doctor's office. The nurse told us the catheter had been put in upside down. She fixed it and gave Mother an appointment to come back in a few days.

By that time, Mother wasn't feeling well. The nurse took the catheter out, but it didn't seem to help. Back home, Mother was sleeping all the time and complained that she was having chills.

When we finally took her temperature and found that she had a fever, we went back to her doctor's office for a third time. The two times before, the actual doctor had never seen her. It had always been the nurse. This time, the doctor came in and immediately told us Mother has a 'Staph' (a *Staphylococcus aureus*) infection. He kept telling her, 'What are you doing here? You should be at the hospital!'

We went directly to the hospital. They admitted her, and within a few days, they said she now had sepsis. That's a really dangerous infection where bacteria get into your blood. They needed to do another surgery to take the sling out because it was infected. But then she got blood clots and had to have another surgery to take those out.

After many, many days in the hospital and lots of vancomycin (an antibiotic) and other drugs, she left the hospital and went to a nursing home to finish her intravenous antibiotic therapy. When she came home, she was still taking lots of medication and needed to use oxygen.

This has been very hard on us, because Mother is only 65 and has never been sick before. I believe this was all caused by Staph and sepsis."

Regards,
Julie's Daughter

I had the opportunity to contact Ms. Rich and share the story as told by her daughter. At the end of her note to me she said:

I tell everyone "Don't have any elective surgery." It's not worth it.

What went wrong? Here was a healthy woman, under age 70, who had elective surgery (meaning it was not an emergency) and ended up with complications. What do you think went wrong?

Let's look at the facts. We know that within 48 hours after a catheter is inserted, it becomes surrounded with bacteria. In this case, Mrs. Rich went back to her doctor's office after 48 hours, and it was determined the catheter was not inserted correctly. The nurse "fixed it" and said to come back in a few days. What probably happened is that "fixing it" moved the catheter in a way that let the surrounding bacteria pass into Mrs. Rich's bloodstream. Because she had just had surgery and her immune system was weak, her body didn't fight off the bacteria. In a short time, she developed sepsis (infection in the blood).

What do you think Julie Rich and her daughter should have done? Here's what I would have told them:

1. Make sure you really need a urinary catheter and that it will be kept in for the shortest time possible.
2. Know the warning signs of infection and act quickly to get medical care.
3. If there is a problem after surgery, insist on speaking with your doctor.
4. Go to the emergency room if your doctor is not available to see you.
5. Never allow a healthcare professional to try to fix a catheter that has been inserted incorrectly. Have them remove the catheter and determine whether it is still needed. If so, a new sterile catheter should be used.

It might also have been a good idea to give Julie an antibiotic after "fixing" her catheter, to prevent bacteria from continuing to multiply in her bloodstream. Fortunately, she survived.

You are an empowered patient, so don't be shy about demanding better care than Julie received.

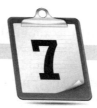

Danger Ahead: Pneumonia
and Other Respiratory Infections

I want you to relax and focus while you read this chapter, so settle into your chair and get comfortable. Now take a deep breath, hold it a while, and very slowly exhale. Feels good, doesn't it?

But just imagine how you'd feel if taking a deep breath became painful and didn't move enough air into your lungs to let you hold your breath for more than a few seconds. Soon you'd start coughing and would feel short of breath even doing normal activities at home. That's what it's like to have pneumonia, a serious bacterial or viral infection of the lower respiratory tract. Pneumonia causes high fever, shaking chills, a cough that produces secretions, shortness of breath, and chest pain that occurs during breathing or coughing.[1]

Each year, about 4 million people living outside of healthcare facilities develop pneumonia, most often during the winter months.[2] This type of pneumonia is called "community acquired" because patients become sick outside of the hospital. It is the most common type of pneumonia. Most people who have community-acquired pneumonia can be treated at home with oral antibiotics and usually begin to feel better in 2 to 3 days. However, elderly people with chronic health problems often need hospital care, and about 10 percent die within 30 days of hospitalization.[3]

GET THE VACCINE!

Infectious disease doctors find that many of these deaths occur because the bacteria that cause pneumonia aren't responding to antibiotic treatment;

in other words, they are resistant to antibiotic treatment. That's especially upsetting, because many people aren't aware that vaccines are available to help prevent pneumonia, and others avoid getting the vaccine because they mistakenly think it is harmful.[4] The pneumococcal pneumonia vaccine is generally recommended for people aged 65 years and older and for adults and some children who have chronic diseases or serious health problems. Just one shot usually provides protection for at least 5 years. Imagine how many pneumonia deaths could be prevented if everyone knew this correct information?

Another important prevention method people often forget is to wash and sanitize their hands frequently. That's especially important during the cold and flu season.

Did You Get a Flu Shot This Year?

Many people develop pneumonia when they have a bad case of the flu, so be sure to get a flu shot (influenza vaccine) every year (unless your doctor advises against it).

Ask your doctor about the pneumonia vaccine, too. Just one shot protects most people for 5 years.

DANGERS AHEAD: HOSPITAL-ASSOCIATED PNEUMONIA

Another category of pneumonia occurs in people who are admitted to a hospital for surgery or other treatments and then develop infections in the lungs and breathing passages (respiratory infections). Medical experts call this "hospital-associated pneumonia" (HAP), meaning that it occurs 48 hours or more after being admitted to a hospital in a patient who had no signs of pneumonia when he or she came to the hospital. It is one of the most common, and most deadly, types of healthcare-associated infections. In fact, studies show that HAP is the second most frequent cause of hospital-associated infections—it accounts for 15–20 percent of all healthcare-associated infections.

HAP occurs most commonly in patients who already have other health problems, such as strokes, or who unable to get out of bed. It is a very serious disease that adds days to a hospital stay, raises the cost of healthcare, and increases patients' risk of dying.[4] I don't want HAP to happen to you! That's why I want you to know what to watch for and what to do to help to prevent pneumonia when you're in the hospital.

Handwashing and sanitizing help to prevent all healthcare-associated infections, especially when you're in the hospital. Unfortunately, that is not enough to protect you from the many risks of HAP. Here are the reasons why. Your nose, mouth, and skin are always exposed to bacteria and viruses floating in the air and landing on surfaces. In hospitals, more bacteria and viruses are floating around, simply because lots of sick people are there. In addition, you may undergo surgery and other hospital procedures that weaken your ability to fight an infection, and you may have incisions or other breaks in the skin that provide new ways for disease-causing germs to enter your body.

With all these risks, it's not surprising that HAP is usually more serious and more difficult to cure than community-acquired pneumonia. Another reason is that hospital germs are often resistant to antibiotics.[1]

Q: How do patients get HAP?

A: The easiest way for pneumonia bacteria to get into your body is via your throat. Outside the hospital that usually happens by breathing in bacteria from the air or by touching a surface that had bacteria on it, and then touching your nose or mouth. Your risks are much greater in the hospital where you may need treatments that can transmit bacteria directly into your airways. One example is a procedure called endotracheal intubation, in which a tube is inserted down the throat and into the breathing passage to help support the patient's ability to breathe. Healthcare workers may also use a suction device to clear away excess mucus from the patient's throat.

During procedures like these, any bacteria that may be on the healthcare worker's hands could spread to the patient's mouth and throat. If the bacteria multiply and become colonized, they can easily pass from the throat into the lower part of a lung and cause pneumonia. This often occurs in patients who can't cough or gag due to weakness or disease, or in patients who take medication that prevents coughing. These problems make it difficult for the body to rid itself of bacteria in the lungs.

Q: Are certain patients more likely to get HAP?

A: Yes, we know that the biggest risks are being older than 70 years, having another serious disease (for example, a chronic pulmonary disease such as emphysema), being malnourished or in a coma, or having stayed in the hospital for a long time. Hospital patients who need to be treated in an intensive care unit have a greatly increased risk of pneumonia.[1]

Q: If I develop pneumonia while I'm in the hospital, does that mean I could die?

A: Unfortunately, a very large number of people develop, and die from, HAP every year. A survey of U.S. hospitals found that over 250,000 children and adults were diagnosed with HAP during 2002, and over 35,000 died. A majority of these pneumonia infections and deaths occurred during treatment in an intensive care unit.[5]

Costs of Care

HAP costs a lot of money to treat. In a recent study of U.S. hospital admissions from 1998 through 2006, researchers checked records for about 79,000 cases of HAP.[6] Over 28,000 of these patients developed pneumonia during hospital treatment that included surgery (requiring an incision):

- They needed to stay in the hospital for an average of 14 extra days.
- The cost for the extra care they required averaged about $46,000 per patient.
- Over 11 percent of the patients died.

For the remaining 51,000 patients who didn't have surgery, pneumonia added hospital time and extra costs, but at a much lower rate. Nevertheless, about 5-10 percent of these patients died. (The lower percentage was for people who had shorter hospital stays.)

WHAT IF YOU NEED A MACHINE TO HELP YOU BREATHE (A VENTILATOR)?

Pneumonia makes it difficult to breathe. That means the level of oxygen in your body may get very low, and you will feel like you can't get enough air. This is a very uncomfortable and scary feeling.

When you're in the hospital, you may have a small device called an *oximeter* (an oxygen saturation monitor) clipped onto your finger that can measure your blood oxygen level. If the level continues to be low, you may be given extra oxygen to breathe. That's easy to do via a tube that clips onto your nostrils or a mask placed over your nose and mouth.

Some people are unable to breathe deeply enough or rapidly enough to maintain a healthy blood oxygen level (a condition called respiratory failure). This is actually a very common problem that affects about 1 percent of people (1 out of 100) who undergo non-emergency abdominal surgery.[7]

Using a ventilator—a machine that helps you breathe—can solve the problem.[8] A ventilator uses pressure to blow air or a mix of air and oxygen into the lungs. The pressure level and "breathing speed" can be adjusted to meet each patient's needs.

Q: How does the breathing machine connect to the person's body?

A: It can connect in two ways, both of which are done under anesthesia (deep sleep), so you won't be awake or feel discomfort:

1. A flexible tube is placed into the patient's mouth and is then moved down past the larynx into the *trachea* (the "wind pipe").This endotracheal tube is mainly used for people who need a breathing machine for only short periods.Tape or a strap that fits around the head holds the tube in place.
2. The second way to connect is via a small surgical opening in front of the neck, through which a tube can be inserted directly into the wind pipe. It's called a tracheotomy tube ("trach" for short).Trach tubes are used mostly for people who need ventilators for long periods or will need their airway protected. Special ties or bands hold the trach in place around the neck.

There are major challenges in having these tubes even though they are necessary to save your life. The tubes pass through your vocal cords, so it makes it difficult or even impossible to speak and eat and limits your ability to move around.

Q: Will I need special care if I'm on a breathing machine?[8]

A: You'll need a special hospital healthcare team of doctors, nurses, and respiratory therapists to keep you safe and healthy while you're on a breathing machine. They will:

- Order chest X-rays and blood tests to check your lungs and monitor the levels of oxygen and carbon dioxide in your bloodstream.
- Place a small tube down your breathing tube on many occasions to remove mucus from your lungs, because you won't be able to do it on your own.
- Feed you nutrient solutions through a tube placed in your nose or mouth that goes into your stomach (feeding tube).
- Check your temperature, blood pressure, lung sounds, and other measures to detect signs that could indicate onset of a dangerous

complication of being on a breathing machine, the development of pneumonia, called ventilator-associated pneumonia.

■ Help you practice brief periods with the breathing machine off to see if you are ready to start breathing on your own.

If You've Had Surgery, You Probably Were on a Breathing Machine (Ventilator)!

The idea of needing a ventilator to breathe is very frightening. You may worry that you'll never recover enough to have it removed. But it may ease your fears to know that, if you've ever been under general anesthesia for surgery, you probably were connected to a ventilator to make sure you kept breathing during the procedure. After surgery, when the medication that puts you asleep (anesthesia) wore off, you began breathing on your own again and the ventilator was disconnected.

Did you know this? Most people don't, because they slept through it. The only clue is the sore throat you probably had after surgery. It was caused by the tube the anesthesiologist inserted into your airway to connect to the breathing machine.

VENTILATOR-ASSOCIATED PNEUMONIA ISN'T INEVITABLE!

Ventilators save many lives, but their use makes it easier for pneumonia bacteria to travel into the lungs, often with bad consequences.[9]

Bacteria that get into your airways are usually removed by coughing. But with a breathing tube in your throat, it's hard to cough. And without coughing, mucus and other secretions accumulate, which gives bacteria a good place to grow. In addition, breathing tubes need periodic removal for cleaning and replacement, which provides an opportunity for bacteria to enter the airways, especially if hygiene practices aren't scrupulously employed. There's also an infection risk due to food and bacteria that may get sucked into the lungs.[9]

With so many opportunities for infection, it's not surprising that many more patients develop breathing machine–related pneumonia, which causes more deaths than HAP. Requiring treatment in an intensive care unit greatly increases the risk of ventilator-associated pneumonia and death. In a study of 880 intensive care patients maintained on ventilators, 132 patients (15 percent) developed ventilator-associated pneumonia. During their hospitalization, 45 percent of these patients died, compared with 32 percent of ventilator patients who had not developed pneumonia.[9]

These facts can be pretty scary but many things can be done so that people won't get pneumonia while they're on a breathing machine. More important, many people who develop ventilator-associated pneumonia do NOT die and DO eventually recover and no longer need a ventilator. I've observed numerous ventilator patients in hospitals in the United States and Europe, and I know what makes the difference:

- Early recognition of pneumonia symptoms
- Immediate administration of the right antibiotics and
- Consistent use of care practices that are supported by scientific research

Ventilator-Associated Pneumonia Does NOT Mean You're Deathly Sick

Studies show that many people recover, get removed from the ventilator, and are discharged from the hospital. Proper care is what makes this possible!

Q: What is the best way to prevent pneumonia when you're on a breathing machine?

A: Not needing mechanical ventilation for a long time is the best way to prevent ventilator-associated pneumonia, but that is often not possible. What is possible is early recognition of potential symptoms of pneumonia. You should be sure that your "vital signs" are checked every day. Are you developing a fever? Is there a decrease in the level of oxygen in your bloodstream (oxygenation)? Do you need more frequent suctioning of secretions? All these symptoms could be early signs of pneumonia.[10]

Speak up and let healthcare workers know if you notice these signs. Also ask if other ventilator patients in your hospital have been contracting pneumonia. That can be a clue that infections are going around. Be sure that your healthcare team reports these concerns to your doctor and lets you know what tests, treatments, or other procedures will be ordered. If no action is taken, be persistent. Patients and their loved ones are part of the healthcare team and should always be asking questions so that they can understand what's being done and question anything that does not seem right.

Q: Can antibiotics prevent ventilator-associated pneumonia?

A: Overuse of antibiotics should always be avoided because of the risk that pneumonia bacteria may become resistant to antibiotic treatment. However, guidelines from the American Thoracic Society and other infection control experts recommend starting "prompt, appropriate, and adequate therapy" with antibiotics if suspected pneumonia symptoms develop. If this is not done, it increases the patient's risk of dying.[10] Similar guidelines from other professional groups like the American College of Chest Physicians say that antibiotic treatment should be started within 12 hours after first detecting symptoms that look like pneumonia.[11]

You know what it means to be empowered, so you or your advocate will need to use those skills to be sure you get good treatment. First, be sure that a sample of mucus from your lungs ("sputum") is sent to a laboratory for examination to identify the specific kind of bacteria that may have infected your airways. Then the doctor can match the drug to the bug. Most hospitals gather data on current infections in their patients, at other local hospitals, and in the local community. These records indicate current levels of resistance within the community to certain antibiotics. Be sure that your doctor refers to this information to help select the right antibiotic that's most likely to work for you.[10]

Match the Drug to the Bug

If you develop pneumonia, taking the right antibiotic is very important. So be sure that a sample of your sputum is sent to a laboratory to identify the specific kind of bacteria that may have infected your airways. That helps your doctor choose the antibiotic that's most likely to cure your infection.

Q: How can I be sure that I'm getting the kind of nursing care that helps to prevent pneumonia and other healthcare-associated infections?

A: It's well known that several nursing care practices can help to prevent ventilator-associated pneumonia.[12] You and your advocates should be aware of them. Before we look at some success stories, you need to know the "four services" the campaign recommended to improve care for ventilator-associated pneumonia[13]:

1. Elevating the head of the patient's bed between 30° and 45°
2. A daily time without sedative medication
3. Daily assessment of readiness for ventilator tube removal
4. Treatment to prevent blood clots in the legs and stomach ulcers

As the patient, you or your advocate can easily monitor these tasks. If they're not being performed, ask why. Remember, you and your loved ones are part of the healthcare team.

WHAT DOES ZERO LOOK LIKE?

I promised to share some success stories. In Texas, Baylor Regional Medical Center at Plano (BRMCP) adopted a "Zero Tolerance" program to eliminate ventilator-acquired pneumonia.[14] They involved their healthcare staff in training sessions, improved their treatment methods based on scientific principles, and even switched to a different brand of breathing tubes that may help to prevent infections. The result: Since March 2007, BRMCP has had no cases of ventilator-associated pneumonia. They estimate that they've saved $150,000 per patient, for a total average direct saving of $3,333,375 from March 2007 through April 2009. That is what zero looks like!

For even more success stories, click on the website for a healthcare improvement organization called The Institute for Healthcare Improvement (http://www.ihi.org). For example, at Contra Costa Regional Medical Center in Martinez, California, the rate of ventilator-associated pneumonia dropped by more than 90 percent, and at Bryan LGH Medical Center in Lincoln, Nebraska, one intensive care unit went 27 months with no cases of ventilator-associated pneumonia. Other improvement stories can be found at http://www.ihi.org/offerings/IHIOpenSchool/resources/Pages/ImprovementStories/default.aspx

---

No Ventilator-Associated Pneumonia?
It Can Be Done!

Several hospitals that participate in quality improvement programs have reduced the number of ventilator-associated pneumonia cases to zero. Others have come close.

It can be done, so choose a hospital that has shown success at preventing pneumonia.

BUNDLE UP FOR SAFETY!

Many hospitals that strive to improve care do even more than the four-step program includes. They make sure that their healthcare workers use a "bundle" of care practices to achieve the best outcome. As I've mentioned before, the benefit comes from tying them all together, which is much more effective than doing just one, two or three, as time permits.[15]

The key components of the ventilator bundle are as follows:

1. Elevation of the head of the bed between 30° and 45°
2. Daily sedation vacations and assessment of readiness to discontinue ventilator use
3. Treatment to prevent stomach ulcer
4. Treatment to prevent leg blood clots
5. Daily oral care with chlorhexidine (an antibacterial oral rinse)

Oral Care

When you're at home, don't you brush your teeth at least twice a day? You'd think that would happen at the hospital, too, but it is often forgotten, especially in the high-tech setting of intensive care units. In one study, for example, researchers at five hospitals observed daily treatment in 253 intensive care unit patients maintained on a ventilator.[16] During an initial 7-day period:

- The only oral care patients received was cleansing with suction swabs.
- None of the patients had their teeth brushed.
- None had moisture applied to the mucous membranes in their mouth.
- Only 32 percent of the patients had oral suctioning done to remove accumulated secretions in the mouth.

But 1 week after healthcare workers were trained in proper oral care:

- Thirty-three percent of the patients had their teeth brushed.
- Sixty-five percent were given swab cleaning.

- Sixty-three percent had moisturizer applied to their oral mucosal tissues.
- Sixty-one percent received suctioning or other care to manage their oral secretions.

Daily oral care helps to decrease plaque and bacterial growth in the oral cavity, so that bacterial colonies don't form and infection doesn't begin. That's important! Here's what studies recommend:

- The proper sequence is to perform oral care every 4 hours with some type of cleanser and to brush the patient's teeth every 12 hours.
- Brushing should be performed with a suctioning toothbrush that attaches to the suction outlet on the wall in the hospital room.
- Oral care should be done by cleaning the patient's mouth with a suction swab soaked in cleansing solution, followed by applying a mouth moisturizer to the whole mouth, including the tongue.

Many hospitals use kits that contain the right equipment needed for oral care. Healthcare workers can use a check list posted in the patient's room and mark when each step is performed. If you don't see oral care equipment or a checklist in the room, ask if hey are available. If not, make one yourself, put it up, and mark down the daily oral care you receive. Part of your role as a member of the healthcare team is to ensure that the proper care is provided, but you can also participate in any of the activities you are comfortable doing.

Oral Care for: _____ *(patient name)*	Room:____					
Oral Care Activity	**Check When Completed**					
	AM			PM		
Brush the teeth using suctioning toothbrush every 12 hours (twice daily, once in the AM and once in the PM)						
Cleanse with antiseptic cleanser or rinse (using suction swab) every 4 hours (up to 3 times in the AM and 3 times in the PM)						
Moisturize oral cavity, including tongue, every time after cleansing (up to 3 times in the AM and 3 times in the PM)						

Example of a daily checklist that family or advocates can use to track the patient's oral care. Share with healthcare workers or post next to the patient's bed.

Elevation of the Head of the Bed

Why is it important for ventilator patients not to lie flat on the bed? Many studies show that lying at a raised angle prevents secretions from gathering in the mouth, where they can enter into the lungs. Preventing this helps to prevent ventilator-associated pneumonia.[17]

Just saying "elevate the head of the bed" doesn't fully explain what must be done. The head of your hospital bed should be raised around 30°. Most people don't remember angle measurements from high school geometry, so they have no idea what 30° would look like. That's why many hospitals place tape markers at 30° on the wall behind the head of a patient's bed, so staff members entering the room can tell if the bed is in the correct position. If these marks aren't on your wall, ask to have them put on. Then monitor the position of your bed and remind healthcare workers to confirm that the head of the bed is at the correct height each time they visit you.

Researchers who monitored bed positioning of mechanically ventilated patients found that the correct head elevation position was not maintained 85 percent of the time, mostly because patients frequently shifted their bodies while in bed.[17] That makes it even more important for the whole healthcare team to strictly follow all the other oral care instructions to ensure the greatest chance of preventing pneumonia.

HANDWASHING SAVES LIVES!

I know I've said it many times already, but I can't say it enough: Hand hygiene is the single most important factor in preventing infections. That's why Job No. 1 for you and your advocate is making sure that every healthcare worker who comes in contact with you sanitizes his or her hands with alcohol gel, or if the hands are soiled, washes them with soap and water.

Healthcare workers are often rushed, so they may forget and put on gloves without washing their hands. They may start providing care for a patient, get interrupted, and then leave the hospital room with gloves on, only to return later and resume treatment without washing or sanitizing their hands again or still wearing the same gloves. You or your advocate *must* insist that all healthcare workers who are in contact with you always remove their gloves and use a hand sanitizer before proceeding.

HEALTHCARE WORKER, DAUGHTER, AND ADVOCATE

Many people have shared their stories with me, and that's how I found Roberta Mikle, RN. Roberta is most impressive with her continued dedication to helping her patients to avoid healthcare-associated infections. Here's what she told me about her father's difficult time in the hospital.

Roberta's Dad

I have been a healthcare professional for more than 25 years, and now I am also a healthcare patient advocate. Why, you may ask? The answer is simple. Throughout my nursing career, I always acted as an advocate for my patients. That often meant going against the usual routine within the work environment and trying new care practices to protect patients.

Then my father, Mickey, developed pneumonia due to resistant bacteria called methicillin-resistant Staphylococcus aureus (MRSA) infection. He almost died because of a lack of basic infection control practices in the hospital where he was treated. That is when the need for a different kind of advocacy hit closer to home. Until that time, I was always advocating for safe care, but I was not specifically focused on preventing infections.

Let me tell you more about what happened to my Dad. He was admitted to the hospital after having a heart problem. The recommended treatment was insertion of a stent to keep his an artery in his heart open. It is a simple procedure that can be performed as an outpatient surgery without any complications. So what went wrong? After the procedure, my Dad needed treatment in the intensive care unit for two days. He was then transferred to a general-care floor for what we assumed would be another few days.

Those few days turned into several weeks. The reason was the terrible cough he developed while he was in the ICU. He coughed up copious amounts of greenish-brown liquid almost continuously—it was unlike anything I had ever seen, and it kept getting worse. Despite all that, he did not need to go on breathing machine and remained out of the ICU after his initial time there. During his extended hospital stay, he remained in a private room.

While my Dad was hospitalized, I began to see what hospital care was like from a patient's perspective. Basic infection control practices were lacking. No one performed the patient care practices that are designed to prevent pneumonia, such as oral care and elevating the head of the bed. In fact, it was only after we brought those needs to the attention of the hospital staff that nurses started turning him in bed and encouraging him to perform deep breathing exercises.

The most important failure was the lack of handwashing. We contacted the infection control department as well as the chief nurse and were told that, 'We are aware of the problems and are working on them.'

After three weeks in the hospital, my Dad was finally discharged. But he needed to go back to the hospital soon after discharge. According to his medical records, cultures from his nostrils and underarms showed that he still had a MRSA infection. He transferred to another hospital where, once again, I saw that infection control practices were not being performed. For example, I saw a respiratory therapist who placed an inhaler in his pocket after a patient used it. Many physicians did not wash their hands after touching a patient, and some healthcare workers would enter data on their computer while standing outside a patient's hospital room, then enter the room without washing their hands.

I realized that asking about handwashing was not going to make an impact on patient care, because there were so many offenders. Instead, I placed a sign on the door to my Dad's hospital room that said, 'Wash hands.' At this point, I needed no additional evidence that it is the responsibility of an advocate (often a family member) to monitor infection control practices together with the healthcare team and take direct action to protect a loved one's health and safety in the hospital.

Some years later, after her father's death, Roberta Mickle mounted an advocacy campaign to improve infection control practices within dialysis facilities in the state of California.

WHAT DOES AN EMPOWERED PATIENT OR LOVED ONE DO?

Roberta's father's case documents two things that we have known for a long time:

- Healthcare workers know the right thing to do, but need to be reminded to do it.
- The foundation for preventing healthcare infections begins with hand hygiene.

Whether you ask hospital caregivers to practice hand hygiene or place a sign on the patient's door asking staff members to wash their hands or use a sanitizer, always remember that it is your right as a patient and/or an advocate to expect the correct care to be provided each time.

Daily Hospital Checklist for Respiratory Illnesses

- ❏ Practice hand hygiene.
- ❏ Check that the head of the patient's bed is correctly elevated to between 30° and 45°.
- ❏ Each day, have the doctor assess the patient's need to continue ventilator use.
- ❏ Make sure the patient receives oral care many times throughout the day when he or she is on a breathing machine.

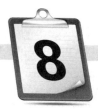

Your Surgery Safety Briefing

Going to the hospital for surgery is a lot like taking a plane trip. The experience is potentially dangerous, but you trust the pilot—or the surgeon—to have the knowledge and expertise to keep you safe. Flight attendants—and healthcare workers in the hospital—will deal with any problems that develop. However, on a plane or in the hospital, you'll need to ring for help and may have to wait until other people's needs are addressed first.

There is one major difference: Before the plane takes off, flight attendants always provide a thorough safety briefing. Every passenger—from small children to adults of all ages and sizes—is taught how to buckle the seatbelts, check for exit locations, and follow emergency floor-path lights leading to each exit. In addition, you're shown how to remove a safety vest from under your seat, put it on correctly, and use the devices that inflate it. Finally, an attendant shows you how to put on an oxygen mask, start the airflow, and then assist a small child or elderly person who needs help doing so. Only then will the plane take off, leaving you at least somewhat prepared to manage emergency situations on your own.

Can you imagine a hospital safety briefing that teaches you how to operate an oxygen mask, or how to help yourself, or assist a friend or loved one, with any aspect of surgical care? Not likely. Hospitals believe you can rely on doctors and nurses to monitor your condition after surgery, and trust them to recognize and manage any signs of trouble.

Are you OK with that? I'm not! This book is designed to make you an empowered, active participant in your care and recovery. How does this apply to surgery? I think every surgery patient deserves a safety briefing, just as much as any airplane passenger. You'll find one here. You'll also find:

- Lists of questions you should ask your surgeon
- Q&A sections to answer your own questions
- A personal story about one man's surgical infection

And that's not all. You probably know that airplane pilots use checklists to make sure they've completed each step needed for a safe takeoff and landing. I think every surgery patient also deserves a checklist. That's coming up, too. So fasten your seatbelt and get ready to take off for the hospital.

YOUR SURGERY SAFETY BRIEFING

"Hospitals are not the safe places we would like them to be." That's the finding issued by members of the Surgical Patient Safety System Collaborative Group in a 2010 medical journal report.[1] The group based their warning on a survey of almost 75,000 patient records from the United States, Canada, the United Kingdom, Australia, and New Zealand. They discovered that nearly 1 out of every 10 people admitted to the hospital experienced an "in-hospital adverse event" (harm resulting from medical care), which resulted in a longer hospital stay or a disability. Fortunately, most of the affected patients experienced only minor disabilities. Unfortunately, 7 percent of the patients died.[2]

Surgery-related problems—especially infections in the part of the body where the surgery took place (surgical site infections or SSIs)—accounted for more than half of all adverse events in this large group of patients.[2] Compared with other surgery patients, people who developed surgical site infections were twice as likely to die, twice as likely to spend time in the intensive care unit, and five times more likely to need another hospitalization after being discharged from the hospital. If you develop a surgical site infection, you're also likely to need four, six, or even more extra days in the hospital, which adds significantly to the cost of care.[3] That's the bad news.

Now for the good news. We know that 40–60 percent of surgical site infections can be prevented by simple practices. Patients like you can play an important role in ensuring that these practices are performed. The Centers for Disease Control and Prevention and other national organizations have developed infection prevention guidelines for both *you* and your healthcare workers.

For example, analysis of the study's 75,000 patient records showed that over 40 percent of all surgical site infections could have been prevented if healthcare workers had followed basic infection control procedures.[2] These "best practice guidelines" include the following[4]:

- Checking that all operating room tools and equipment are sterile
- Administering preventive antibiotics
- Making sure surgical sponges and needles aren't left inside the body

Prevent Surgical Infections!

If you develop a surgical site infection, you have a greater risk of needing intensive care and a longer stay in the hospital. You might even die.

The good news is that you can help to protect yourself from getting an infection. Reminding healthcare workers to wash or sanitize their hands is No. 1 on your infection protection checklist.

In a study at eight hospitals from around the world, surgical complications occurred in 18 percent of patients *before* operating room checklists were used, compared with only 12 percent *after* introduction of surgical safety checklists. Death rates dropped from about 4 out of every 100 patients to between 1 and 2 out of every 100 patients.[5]

That's the benefit of using checklists in the operating room. But the study of 75,000 surgery patients I mentioned previously showed that only 41 percent of all adverse events occurred in the operating room; 25 percent occurred in patients' rooms.[2] That's why many hospitals insist that healthcare workers follow lists of safety procedures (referred to as "bundles") targeted to each stage of your care[6]:

- Before your surgery ("pre-op")
- During your surgery ("operative")
- After your surgery ("post-op")
  and even
- After you leave the hospital ("post-discharge")

Of course, just telling people what they should do doesn't guarantee they'll always do it. Typically, healthcare workers do only some checklist items while other items get neglected. You've already learned that many medical professionals forget to wash or sanitize their hands, even in the intensive care unit. It may be up to you to remind them, especially after surgery. That's why you can't just "sit back, relax, and enjoy the flight," as you do on a plane.[7]

Infections can start at any stage of your surgical care, but you can play an active role in preventing them. Yes, you really can help yourself. This chapter will show you how.

PRE-OP *PREPARATION*

The American College of Surgeons, the organization that certifies surgeons' professional competence, wanted to know how much time and effort people spend preparing for surgery, compared with other important life events. Here's what their 1,000-person survey showed:

- Changing jobs (10 hours spent, on average)
- Buying or leasing a new car (8 hours)
- Planning a $1,000 vacation (4 hours)
- Researching their surgical procedure or their surgeon (*just 1 hour!*)

Even more surprising, about one out of three Americans in the survey who had undergone surgery didn't even check their surgeon's credentials beforehand.[8] Was the surgeon board certified? Did he or she have specific training in the specialty involved in the procedure, that the patient was having? These details, and several others, are important factors in choosing a qualified surgeon. An excellent resource that gives information on how to choose a hospital or doctor is Consumer Reports at http://www.consumerreports.org/health/doctors-hospitals/hospitals/choosing-a-hospital/best-doctor.htm

Questions to Ask

By reading this book, you've already become an empowered patient, so I know you'll spend more than an hour choosing a qualified surgeon and a good hospital, and determining how much of your cost is covered by insurance. However, if you need emergency surgery, there's no time to make advance plans. So while you're feeling well, take time to ask which major hospital in your area your doctor would recommend for emergency care and which local surgeons are highly qualified to perform procedures you may need. Share this information with someone who can speak for you if you get too sick or injured to speak for yourself.

Good News!

Starting in 2012, patients and consumers have additional data to study before choosing a doctor or hospital. Our government will now make available to employers, insurance companies, and consumer groups data from Medicare claims that tell how often a surgeon performs a procedure and how often problems such as preventable complications result. Prior to this, only data from patients *not* on Medicare were available for comparision, which was not a good representation of all patients and doctors given the large number of patients that are on Medicare.

Doctors will be identified, but not patients, making it easy for consumers to find this information before they are hospitalized. These data will also allow for reports on many specialists as well. The first consumer reports should be available at https://www.cms.gov/medicare-coverage-database/.

In nonemergency situations, your pre-op preparation should also include meeting with the surgeon before you check into the hospital. You'll want to ask the following[8,9]:

- What will happen during my surgery? The surgeon may use pictures or videos to explain things to you.
- What complications could occur and what would be done to manage them?
- What is the risk of infection and what will be done to prevent it (such as precautionary antibiotic treatment)?
- What do I need to do to get ready for my surgery? Many surgeons provide a written instruction sheet telling you what tests you need before the day of surgery, whether you should shower beforehand, or if you should fast or discontinue taking certain medicines.
- What special care, tests, or therapy will I need in the hospital after surgery?

- How long will I have to stay in the hospital?
- What kind of care will I need during recovery at home or in a nursing home?
- What is my role as I recover from surgery?

During your pre-op visit, the surgeon will also ask you questions about your general health, allergies, nutrition, and medications you're taking. That's because people with some medical conditions are more likely to develop surgical site infections and may need preventive care.

Q: How do I know whether I have a higher risk of getting a surgical site infection?

A: We know that the following personal factors can increase your risk of developing an infection after surgery[10]:

- Diabetes
- Cigarette smoking
- Use of steroids
- Being overweight
- Advanced age
- Poor nutrition
- Cancer and immune system diseases
- Paralysis or limited mobility
- Prolonged hospital stay before surgery
- Already having an infection

PRE-OP *PREVENTION*

Preventing infections begins before you have your surgery. One important prevention step is to take control of the conditions on the risk list. For example, if you have diabetes, be sure you're maintaining healthy blood sugar levels. If you smoke, have a poor diet, or weigh too much, do something about it before scheduling your surgery.

Your surgeon may also tell you to reduce bacteria levels on your skin by bathing with an antiseptic soap containing chlorhexidine before you go to the hospital.[11] You can purchase this over the counter in the drug store under the brand names such as Betasept, Calgon Vesta, Chlorostat, Hibiclens, and others. However, don't shave near the area where you'll have a surgical incision. Shaving was a standard procedure for many years, but we now know that shaving can cause small nicks in the skin that let bacteria get into the body.[12]

Of course, you can't control everything by yourself. For example, some people are unknowingly colonized with methicillin-resistant *Staphylococcus aureus* (MRSA) bacteria in their nostrils, even though they haven't yet developed an infection. To prevent the spread of these dangerous bacteria, many hospitals require incoming patients to have nasal samples cultured for *S. aureus*. Some patients found to be infected may be treated with a nasal antibiotic ointment.[13]

Five Steps to Take Before Surgery

1. If you have diabetes, maintain healthy blood sugar levels. Check your A1c level, make sure it is less than 7 percent. (Hemoglobin A1c is a measure of your average blood sugar level during the prior 2–3 months.)
2. If you smoke, quit now!
3. If you're overweight, improve your diet and get more exercise to help burn more calories.
4. Do not shave the area where you'll have surgery.
5. If you have been told you have a MRSA infection, inform your surgeon.

Q: Are some surgeries more likely than others to result in an infection?

A: Yes. We know that infection risks are higher when surgery is performed on sites that we call *dirty*—like the bowel or a ruptured appendix. When a surgical procedure lasts more than 2 hours or requires blood transfusions during the operation, the risk of developing an infection is also increased.[14]

IN THE OPERATING ROOM

Whether or not you develop an infection depends not just on your health condition and your prevention efforts, but mostly on what happens in the operating room and in your hospital room. You won't be awake during surgery, but beforehand, you can watch for infection risks or errors, and speak up if you have concerns.

For example, if a healthcare worker tries to shave you with a razor, ask why. As you just read, preoperative shaving isn't recommended anymore. If hair needs to be removed, it should be done immediately before surgery, using a hair clipper.[15]

Before your surgery starts, a healthcare worker should check your name and ask you to confirm where the surgery will be performed. Left arm or right arm? Left leg or right leg? Chest or abdomen? According to the best practice guidelines, that person should put a mark on the correct site or ask you to do it yourself. If this is not done, then ask to speak with either your doctor or a member of the surgical team.

This may seem foolish to you, but operating on the wrong patient or on the wrong body part ("site") happens more often than you think. In a study of medical errors from 2002 to June of 2008, physicians reported 25 wrong-patient incidents and 107 wrong-site incidents.[16] These errors are known as "never events," because they're so serious and so easily prevented that they should *never* occur. Make sure they never happen to you by insisting that the presurgery practice guidelines are followed.

Q: Will I be given an antibiotic before my surgery?

A: Use of antibiotics reduces the risk of infections in many surgical procedures. If your doctor tells you that you will receive antibiotics, the important question to ask is how he or she will ensure that the antibiotic is *administered within 60 minutes before the first incision* is made.[12] The reason for the 60-minute window is that having the most antibiotic in your system at the time the incision is made will ensure that you are protected from bacteria that might get into the wound. For some antibiotics, administration 30–60 minutes before surgery is more effective than administration during the final 30 minutes.[17]

We know that if an antibiotic is given after surgery or too long before surgery, it has no effect in preventing infection. It is like closing the barn door after the horse is out. This may seem like something you'd assume that every doctor would know. Unfortunately, despite the presence of evidence and guidelines, the fact is that 25–50 percent of the time, the antibiotic is administered at the wrong time, at the wrong dose, or not at all.[18,19] So if your doctor told you that an antibiotic would be given, remember to ask about it right before your surgery.

Don't Count on Doctors to Remember Everything!

Research shows the time you receive an antibiotic before surgery is very important in preventing an infection. So before you're wheeled into the operating room, be sure to ask if, and when, you'll be given an antibiotic.

Q: Will my blood sugar level be monitored before and after surgery?

A: As I mentioned before, if you are diabetic, your risk of a surgical site infection is greater than that of a non-diabetic person. In addition to the stress of having surgery, you may be told to stop taking your usual diabetes medications before surgery and to alter your normal meal schedule, all of which can cause an increase in blood glucose (sugar). Research has shown that non-diabetics also may have an upswing in blood glucose during and after surgery. According to a recent study, this excessively elevated blood sugar (*hyper*glycemia) may be the No. 1 risk factor for surgical site infections.[20] (Note that "hyper" means high or above; "hypo" means low or below.) Make sure your hemoglobin A1c level is lower than 7 percent.

Whether or not you have diabetes, the message here is to make sure your blood glucose is checked before and after most types of major surgery, so appropriate medication can be given if necessary. Blood sugar monitoring should continue for 48 hours post-surgery, because high blood glucose levels continue to increase your risk of developing an infection.

How high is too high? Until recently, surgeons aimed to keep patients' blood sugar levels below 200 mg/dL, the American Diabetes Association's recommended level.[21] However, recent studies show that more intensive glucose control—to levels below 140 mg/dL—may be needed to prevent infections.[20,21] Ask your surgeon what's best for your type of surgery and your personal health history.

Q: I've heard that it's important to be kept warm during and after surgery. Is that true?

A: People get cold during surgery for two main reasons: operating rooms are kept at cool temperatures and surgical anesthesia interferes with the body's temperature-regulating mechanisms.[22] Studies have shown that experiencing hypothermia (body temperature less than 96.8°F) during surgery can increase the risk of a surgical site infection and that patients who are kept warm to maintain normal temperature have lower rates of infection (especially during colon and rectal surgery).[23] We also know that for any type of surgery, the occurrence of serious heart problems can be reduced by maintaining a normal body temperature.

On the basis of these reports, many physicians and medical organizations recommend monitoring patients' body temperatures during surgery, and "warming" anyone whose temperature falls below 96.8°F (this is purposely lower than 98.6°F, the usual "normal"). For example, hospitals throughout the United States participate in the Surgical Care Improvement Project (SCIP), a national quality partnership dedicated to reducing the rate of surgical complications. SCIP recommends warming for colorectal surgery patients.

However, a recent analysis of patient records for 398 SCIP member hospitals failed to show that maintaining normal body temperature during surgery decreased post-operative infections in these patients.[24] A separate study at one SCIP member hospital also found no evidence that maintaining normal temperature during colorectal and other surgeries reduced the risk of surgical site infections.[25] Current recommendations from the U.S. Centers for Disease Control do not include warming.[12]

Whether or not to control surgery patients' temperatures is still unresolved. Ask your surgeon if warming is used in your hospital. If so, it may be as simple as increasing the temperature in the operating room, having you wear a hat and booties during surgery, or putting a warmed blanket over you, especially before surgery, to help you store the heat in your body. Body temperature can also be maintained by administering warmed intravenous fluids during surgery.

Q: Are there any last-minute questions I should ask the surgeon?

A: Yes, there is one important question to ask, and it's sure to surprise you. Most hospitals have rules that limit the number of hours doctors can work during the 24-hour day, because fatigue and sleep deprivation seriously impair performance. In fact, one study showed that when surgeons got less than 6 hours of sleep before a non-emergency, daytime operation, their patients had a significant 83 percent increase in their risk of suffering complications.[26]

Some experienced surgeons might be able to do an excellent job even when they're half asleep, but would you want them to? I think surgeons should tell you if they're sleep deprived, so you can decide whether or not to go ahead with the scheduled operation. Their full disclosure is necessary for you to give truly informed consent to undergo a surgery. After all, you're about to be put to sleep, but you wouldn't want your surgeon to fall asleep, too.

POST-SURGERY INFECTION RISKS

Your operation is over, and everything went well. But it's still important to watch out for infections. Here's why. Our skin does an amazing job of protecting us from infections, but as you read in the previous chapters, even a small cut can let dangerous germs invade the body. Now just imagine how easy it is for germs to get through the much larger opening of your surgical incision. Although surgery is performed in an operating room under sterile conditions, using sterile instruments and supplies, you may think your surgical site couldn't become infected. Actually, there's no way to totally eliminate bacteria. You can get them from two sources[27]:

1. **Endogenous bacteria:** These are the bacteria you already have on your skin. We think of them as *part of the patient*. Even if your skin is thoroughly cleaned with antibacterial agents, some endogenous bacteria will remain. When an incision is made, these bacteria can enter the body.

   You also have endogenous bacteria inside your body. For example, bacteria are always present *inside* the large intestines and other organs without causing any trouble. However, if they spill *out* during surgery, into spaces like the abdominal cavity (the peritoneum), serious infections can occur.

2. **Exogenous bacteria:** These are bacteria from sources *outside the patient*. Sources can include air in the operating room, and contaminated surgical instruments and devices such as hip or knee replacements that are put in during surgery. Even the surgical silk sutures or metal staples used to close the incision can carry bacteria through your skin. Bacteria attach to the surfaces of these objects, then quickly multiply and produce toxins that help them survive and cause infection.

Q: I almost never get infections, even colds. So why is everyone warning me that I could get a surgical site infection?

A: After surgery, exogenous bacteria sources surround you, including environmental surfaces, medical equipment brought into your room, and people with infections who may be sharing the hospital room with you. Usually, your own immune system can fight these infections, but when you undergo surgery, your immune system is weakened. Bacteria take advantage of this opportunity to invade and cause infections.

Q: How will I know if I have a surgical site infection?

A: Surgical site infections occur in the area of the incision. It's normal to see some slight swelling or bruising around your closed incision right after surgery, but be on the alert for changes and other signs and symptoms of an infection, including

- Redness at the site of the wound
- Swelling
- Heat (feeling warm to the touch)
- Tenderness or pain
- Drainage (bloody, pus-like fluid)
- Odor

If you see anything suspicious, or if you develop a fever, tell your healthcare workers immediately. If you think the problem isn't being managed well, ask to speak directly with your doctor. Catching and treating an infection in the early stages can make a real difference in your recovery. Waiting could be disastrous.

Immediately after surgery is the time when being watchful and willing to ask questions can make a real difference in protecting yourself from developing a surgical site infection. The first 48 hours are especially important, because your wound (the closed incision) has not had time to start healing yet.[23] You could be too weak or unable to help yourself at that point, so call on an advocate in advance to be with you after surgery.

Why You Need an Advocate

Immediately after surgery, you may be weak, tired, and not very alert.

That's why you need an advocate to stay with you at all times.

So be sure to make advance arrangements with a loved one or friend to be with you and speak for you as an advocate.

PREVENTION TIPS

As I've told you in almost every chapter of this book, the single most important thing you and your advocate can do to prevent infections is to make sure that you and all visitors and healthcare workers who come in contact with you washes their hands with soap and water or a sanitizer.

Bacteria and viruses can also spread via sneezing and coughing, so always cover your mouth when you sneeze or cough, and then wash or sanitize your hands. Ask people who come in contact with you to do the same.

When post-op surgical site infections occur, it's often the result of poor infection control practices and poor hand hygiene practices.[28] Protect yourself! If you see something, say something! Remind healthcare workers and visitors to wash or sanitize their hands.

Wound Care

Hand hygiene reminders are particularly important when it comes to protecting your wound from germs. For example:

- Your bandages should be changed and/or your wound area cleaned frequently. Be sure this is done using sterile practices. Seeing the healthcare worker open bandages or equipment wrappings marked "sterile" is a good sign.
- Before any healthcare worker touches your wound area, be sure they wash or sanitize their hands first, and then use sterile procedures when putting on surgical gloves. If you don't actually see healthcare workers wash or sanitize, ask if they did.
- During your hospital stay, don't touch your wound area and bandages, and don't let family or friends do so either. (Before you go back home, you may be told how to do this safely to help care for yourself.)

Daily Examinations

A doctor or other healthcare worker should examine you every day, to check for signs of infection or other problems.[23] If it doesn't happen, say something! Ask about the schedule for daily examinations and then, if you notice the healthcare team is not adhering to that schedule, remind them of the routine they informed you about.

- Examination of your surgical site should start within 24–48 hours after surgery.
- Any healthcare worker who examines your wound should be experienced in infection prevention. Ask the person about his or her training in wound care.

■ The antibiotic medication you were given before or during surgery should be stopped after 24 hours, unless your doctor says additional use is needed. If your healthcare workers continue to give you antibiotics, ask why.

One more thing: If your hospital room is shared by other patients, ask them if they have any infections. If they do, this may suggest that an infection is going around, and you could be the next one to get it. Talk with your doctor and ask if you should be moved to a safer room.

IT'S TIME TO GO HOME!

Even if you're not moved to another hospital room, your next move could be out of the hospital. Due to cost cutting and insurance limitations, hospital stays are now much shorter than in the past. Patients are often discharged only 1 or 2 days after surgeries that used to require a week or more of recovery time in the hospital.

That means you'll be on your own—or with just a family member to help—to change your bandages, manage your pain medicines, and deal with any medical problem that arises, including a surgical site infection. These infections generally occur within 30 days after surgery, so you're likely to be back home if and when infection symptoms appear.[29]

In one study of 4,500 surgery patients, 89 people (about 2 percent) developed surgical site infections within 8 weeks after returning home. Compared with patients who stayed healthy, the infected patients needed significantly more outpatient doctor or emergency room visits, X-rays, home health aide services, and hospital readmissions, at an average total cost of over $5,000. In contrast, the other healthy patients cost "only" about $1,700 during that time period.[29]

Before You're Discharged

As the study showed, surgical site infections are not only uncomfortable, dangerous, and depressing, they're also time consuming and costly to treat. So I don't want you to be like the study's unfortunate 2 percent! Start protecting yourself by speaking with a discharge planner before you leave the hospital. Here's what you need to find out[30]:

■ Don't leave the hospital until you are given detailed instructions on how to care for your wound and manage other problems that could arise.

- Be sure you understand every one of the home care activities that are needed. You should be given written information to help you remember what to do. Ask questions *before* you leave for home.
- Make sure to ask about bathing. If you're told to use any specific products, ask where you can get them or if the hospital will supply them.
- If you need home health services or medical equipment, get help to obtain them *before* you leave the hospital.
- Get the name and telephone number of a healthcare representative from the hospital who you can call if you have questions or need help while you're back home.
- Schedule an appointment for a follow-up visit.

Managing Home Care

In the hospital, healthcare workers checked your wound and changed your dressings. Now it's up to you to be vigilant in checking your wound every day. The most important thing to remember is to always wash or sanitize your hands before and after touching the bandages and the surgical site!

I don't expect you to remember every one of the many infection prevention tips you read about in this chapter, so I made a checklist for you on page 133. Pay special attention to the instructions about protecting your wound from germs.

Despite your good care, the wound area may develop swelling, redness, oozing, or other signs of infection. Call your doctor immediately if you suspect a problem.

- *Do not settle for speaking with a member of the office staff.* Ask to speak with the doctor. If the doctor is not immediately available, ask to speak to a nurse (instead of an office staff person) and explain that you do need to speak with the doctor that day.
- Provide a telephone number where you can be reached at any time, either at home or via a cell phone.

This can be a very difficult situation, because doctors' office staff members often act as gatekeepers and try to save doctors from being interrupted by unimportant phone calls. As a result, patients may be shy about demanding to speak with a doctor. I assure you that using the technique above will convey a sense of urgency, so your message will be quickly passed along to your doctor.

If you don't get a return call within a few hours, be sure to call again before office hours end that day. If you have signs of an infection, you cannot afford to wait until your scheduled post-operative visit. Be persistent!

DR. McGUCKIN, MEDICAL DETECTIVE

In previous chapters, you've read about some of the people I've met who developed serious, often preventable, healthcare acquired infections. The risk of these infections is especially high following surgery, and the damage is often tragic. When that happens, victims frequently sue the doctor or hospital. That's where I come in.

Here's what happened to a man I'll call Mr. X. At age 73, he needed surgery to remove a brain tumor of the left auditory nerve (the 8th vestibulocochlear nerve). It wasn't emergency surgery, and he had no previous or current medical conditions, so he was in the low-risk category for infection.

After surgery, Mr. X did well at first, but a few days later he developed a fever. Because his surgery was in the head area, doctors decided to take a culture of his spinal fluid to check for infection. They were right. The spinal fluid contained many white blood cells, a definite sign of infection. Looking at the fluid under a microscope, they saw a dangerous kind of rod-shaped bacteria (gram negative rods).

Checking further, they took a sample of fluid draining from Mr. X's head wound. Culture tests of the fluid identified the bacteria as *Klebsiella*. This suggested that the infection had started in his head wound and then spread to his spinal fluid.

Unfortunately, the infection continued to spread, causing meningitis, an infection of the membranes covering the brain and spinal cord. As a result, Mr. X developed weakness both arms and both legs (quadriparesis). How serious is this? It's related to quadriplegia, in which all four limbs are totally paralyzed.

When Mr. X filed a lawsuit, I was called in to investigate why and how he became infected. As usual, I started by reviewing hospital records for the 3 months around the time period Mr. X was hospitalized. I discovered that 12 other patients who were treated in the same intensive care unit as Mr. X also developed infections with the same *Klebsiella* bacteria. Clearly, there was an infection outbreak in that unit, and Mr. X was unlucky enough to wind up there.

Based on experience, I didn't need to dig too deeply to figure out how the infection had spread. As often happens, bacteria from the first infected patient or patients came in contact with equipment and surfaces in the intensive care unit. Most probably, new patients got infected through cross contamination—that is, transfer of bacteria from one person or object to another person. That happens when people don't wash or sanitize their hands! My conclusion: Infection prevention guidelines were not followed. Healthcare workers were not using basic hygiene practices and possibly were not properly sterilizing equipment in the intensive care unit. If the hospital hadn't been checking for infections, the only way to know was when Mr. X and other patients got sick. No wonder his case landed in court!

Q: Could Mr. X have done anything to prevent this terrible outcome?

A: The single most important thing he—or any patient, including *you*—could do is ask the surgeon if there were any outbreaks of infection or an unusual number of cues that infections were occurring in the hospital unit where he would be moved to after his surgery.

Q: What obligation did his surgeon have to tell him about this?

A: Remember what you read about informed consent? In order to give consent, a patient must be fully informed about all relevant facts. Mr. X's surgeon should have told him about the infection cluster. If the doctor didn't know about it, the hospital should have known and should have informed all their doctors.

Surgical Site Infection Prevention Checklist

When you go the hospital for surgery, you want to go home feeling better than when you came in. Avoiding surgical site infections can help to make that happen. Here are my "Top 10" steps you and your healthcare workers should take to prevent those infections:

1. Take a shower or bath the night before, and the morning of, your surgery using a chlorhexidine cleanser, available at your local pharmacy.

2. Ask about pre-operative antibiotics and be sure they are administered within one hour before the first surgical incision is made.
3. Make sure your surgical site will not be shaved.
4. Ask to have your blood sugar tested before surgery. If the surgery is elective, discuss your current hemoglobin A1c level with your doctor.
5. Ask that your body temperature be monitored and controlled during and after surgery.
6. If you were given antibiotic medication during surgery and are still receiving it after 24 hours, ask why it has not been discontinued.
7. Make sure that you and every visitor and healthcare worker who comes in contact with you washes or sanitizes their hands before approaching your bed.
8. Know the signs and symptoms of surgical site infection.
9. Monitor your wound and any intravenous catheters daily for signs of infection.
10. Contact your doctor if you have any concerns.

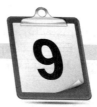

Preventing Bloodstream Infections

The best way to understand bloodstream infections is to imagine taking a lightning-fast ride through your body's bloodstream. If you look at the veins on your hands and arms, you might have trouble imagining how to get inside for the ride. That question was answered in a 1960s science fiction movie called *Fantastic Voyage*, in which medical experts shrank themselves and their submarine down to microscopic size so they could be injected into a scientist's bloodstream. Their biggest problem was surviving the body's immune defense system that works to kill any invaders.

Although you can't shrink yourself down that small, here's how to picture the ride those microscopic experts took. An average 150-pound man has about 5½ liters of blood in his body (picture three 2-liter bottles of soda). The heart is so powerful that it pumps all of this blood in a complete circuit through the entire body in just a little over one minute.[1]

During that minute, blood cells bring oxygen, nutrients, and other compounds to every organ and body part. If invaders—bacteria and viruses, for example—get into the bloodstream, a single one-minute ride could spread serious infections throughout the body. And then the ride continues, circulating those germs about 60 times every hour, throughout the day. Infection-fighting white blood cells will kill many of the invaders, but may not get all of them.

Obviously, your hospital stay won't include a fast ride around your bloodstream in a microscopic submarine. But you may need to have an intravenous catheter (a thin, flexible tube) inserted through your skin into a vein, so fluids and medications can be delivered directly into your bloodstream. In the chapter about urinary catheters, you read about infection risks from bacteria that travel along the catheter into the bladder. As you can guess, the risk of infection is even greater with a catheter that's inserted directly into your bloodstream.

But here's the good news: In many hospitals, your chance of developing a catheter-related bloodstream infection is exactly ZERO! That's thanks to the widespread use of simple checklists for easy measures to prevent catheter-related bloodstream infections. You need to know what these simple measures are, and how you can use your own checklist to make sure healthcare workers keep you infection free. So keep reading, as I take you on a ride through a catheter and into your bloodstream.

IS THERE A CATHETER IN YOUR FUTURE?

Urinary catheters use a long, thin, flexible tube that drains urine out of the bladder and down into a plastic bag. Bloodstream catheters—better known as intravenous lines or "IVs"—have a similar flexible tube. One end of the tube is inserted it into a vein. The longer end of the tube remains outside the body and is used to convey fluids or medications down into the vein. A locking device opens and closes the tube, as needed.

Q: Will I need to have an IV?

A: When you're in the hospital, there may be times when you need fluid or medications on a continuous basis. That's why almost every adult admitted to the hospital will have a short IV catheter inserted, usually in the hand or in the lower arm. It's taped in place. We call it a peripheral catheter, which means it's not entering a central part of your body.

Q: How is the IV put in?

A: Before the IV is inserted, your skin will be cleaned with an antiseptic that kills germs around the area where the IV goes in. Then, an elastic band is placed around your upper arm and drawn tight to reduce blood flow into your lower arm. Next, a hollow needle that's attached to the catheter tube is inserted into your vein—this may cause pain, but it's over quickly. The needle is then removed, leaving the small end of the catheter tube inside the vein, with the longer end extending outside your arm. Transparent tape is applied to hold everything in place and to permit easy examination of the area. Now, the elastic band is released and your blood again flows normally.

Q: How does the peripheral IV work?

A: A device at the outside end of the catheter nearest to your skin can be opened to let healthcare workers take blood samples out for testing.

That way, you won't need to have a needle stuck into your vein every time a sample is needed.

The long tube outside your body is usually connected to a plastic bag filled width fluid that's hooked on a stand above your head. Gravity helps the fluid drip slowly through the catheter to deliver glucose (sugar water), antibiotics, or other medications into your bloodstream.

Q: How long will I need to have a catheter?

A: Peripheral IVs are meant for short-term use, generally 72 hours or less.[2,3] If you need longer intravenous treatment or if the fluids and medications you require can't be administered via a peripheral line, you may need a central venous catheter. I'll tell you more about central lines later in the chapter.

Q: Can I get an infection from a peripheral catheter?

A: Any invasive device can be a cause of infection. All catheters are considered invasive because they are inserted through a break in your skin—that's what invasive means in medical terms. The opening through your skin and into a vein is a perfect entry way for bacteria, but that does *not* mean you'll get an infection.

Here's why. Bacteria can get into your bloodstream even when you brush your teeth. We call this bacteremia. But your body's immune system goes into action to kill the bacteria so you don't develop an infection. The same thing usually happens when you have a peripheral catheter. Because both the catheter needle and the tube that goes into the vein are narrow and they're inserted under sterile conditions, the initial risk of bacteria getting into the bloodstream is low. The insertion site is covered with tape, which also helps, as does keeping the area clean and changing dressings under sterile conditions. The peripheral IV is usually kept in place for less than 72 hours; the shorter the time, the lower the risk of infection.

Knowing all this, you won't be surprised to learn that peripheral catheters are responsible for only about 10 percent of all healthcare-associated bloodstream infections. Most of the remaining 90 percent are due to central venous catheters, which we'll talk about next.[4]

Because of that 10 percent risk, you and your healthcare workers still need to watch for signs that an infection may be developing, such as:

- Discomfort or leakage at the catheter site, which may mean that the catheter tip has slipped out of place

- Redness, swelling, or warmth
- Fever

Q: Is there anything I can do to prevent an infection while I have an IV?

A: Your healthcare workers know the "bundle" of preventive measures they should use, but it's up to you to be sure that your IV care includes all of those measures. Missing even one prevention guideline can outweigh the benefits of other prevention measures that have been taken.

The basic steps included in the preventive care "bundle" for peripheral venous catheters usually include[2,5]:

- ■ Handwashing and other hygiene precautions to ensure sterile conditions at the time the catheter is inserted.
- ■ Cleansing the skin with an antiseptic immediately prior to the catheter insertion.
- ■ Daily examination of the catheter site to see whether a change of dressing or catheter adjustment is needed or if any signs of infection are present.
- ■ Frequent flushing of the catheter to prevent blood clots that interfere with fluid inflow.
- ■ Changing tubing, filters, and other equipment by 72 hours after insertion of the catheter.
- ■ Daily physician review to determine whether the catheter is still necessary.
- ■ Removal of the catheter under sterile conditions, often done prior to 72 hours, but after a longer period if the patient still needs it.

Your being alert and watchful can make a big difference when you have a catheter, as was shown in a recent study. Doctors at a large hospital in Dublin, Ireland, asked 178 patients who had a peripheral venous catheter whether they were aware of the reason they needed it. Surprisingly, 67 patients had no idea why the catheter was put in. Compared to "aware" patients, these unaware individuals were about seven times more likely to have a catheter still in place when it was no longer needed (for example, when administration of intravenous fluids or antibiotics had already been stopped). To prevent infections, catheters should be removed as soon as conditions permit.[5]

The Dublin researchers were so alarmed by their findings, they created a patient information booklet that's now given to every patient in their hospital who has a peripheral venous catheter. Their booklet highlights the ways patients can play a role in preventing infections, including alerting healthcare workers when a catheter should be removed. That's what reading this book is doing for you.

Now that you know about important infection control measures for peripheral catheters, use the checklist (below) to help you remind the hospital staff if they aren't providing important, correct care.

IV Checklist

When you have a peripheral IV line in place, you should *not* develop an infection; that is, if healthcare workers follow all the recommended prevention guidelines. If you aren't getting these care measures, speak up! Here's what to watch for:

1. When someone approaches your bed to insert a peripheral line, ask why you need one and when it will be removed. If you don't understand the explanation, ask to speak to your doctor or a nursing supervisor.
2. At the time the peripheral catheter is inserted, the healthcare worker should wash his/her hands first, before putting on gloves, and should then place a sterile blue pad under your arm.
3. Next, the skin area should be cleansed with an antiseptic solution.
4. The catheter area should be checked every day for signs of infection or other problems. If dressing changes or adjustments are needed, healthcare workers should first clean their hands, put on gloves, and use an antiseptic solution to clean the area.
5. Healthcare workers should do a daily review to perform required adjustments and to determine if you still need to have the peripheral catheter.
6. If you are not alert or well enough to watch and remind healthcare workers about these procedures, be sure to have an advocate with you during your hospital stay.

WILL YOU NEED A CENTRAL VENOUS CATHETER?

There are many types of catheters, some that are inserted into a vein for temporary use, such as the peripheral IVs already discussed, and other catheters that are designed for long-term use. For example, people with kidney disease who need dialysis treatments may have a permanent catheter inserted into a large vein, with a "port" just under the skin through which dialysis solutions can be administered.

Another type of long-term use catheter, known as a central venous catheter ("central line"), is usually placed in the neck, chest, or groin area, in a large vein that carries blood rapidly toward the heart. Fluids or medications delivered through the central line immediately enter these major blood vessels, so they take effect quickly.

Q: Why do people need a central venous catheter?

A: Central venous catheters are vitally important for seriously ill people in the intensive care unit, where they may need rapid administration of blood, large amounts of fluid, or frequent doses of medication for pain, infection, cancer, or heart problems. Central lines are also used for administration of nutritional solutions and as an access site for medical tests such as heart catheterization.[6,7] An increasing number of people outside the hospital (outpatients) now have central venous catheters inserted to provide continuous access to veins for administration of antibiotics, at-home dialysis, and other therapies.

Q: How are central lines different from peripheral IVs?

A: Central venous catheters are much larger in diameter than those used for peripheral IVs. They're also inserted into much larger blood vessels, such as the internal jugular vein on the side of the neck, the femoral vein in the groin area, or the subclavian vein below the collar bone area in the upper chest.

In a subclavian line, central venous catheters can be quite complex, sometimes providing several compartments (lumen). For example, a catheter of this type may have three places for fluids to get into your body, which is called a triple-lumen catheter and is useful for administering different medications at the same time, as is often needed for antibiotics or cancer chemotherapy drugs. Sutures ("stitches") hold the equipment in place at the top and the bottom.[8]

Q: Central lines look scary. Isn't it dangerous and painful to have one put in?

A: Because they're complex and they're placed in deep veins that aren't easy to see, inserting central lines correctly can be difficult. Be sure to ask if the person doing the insertion is experienced in placing central lines like yours. If not, wait until a more experienced person is available!

Healthcare workers who have done central line insertions many times know how to prevent pain with a local anesthetic ("numbing medicine") and how to avoid bleeding and damage to blood vessels and other nearby structures. For example, if the catheter needle misses the vein, it could pierce your lung and cause it to collapse (a serious but treatable condition called pneumothorax). However, when everything is done right, the catheter can remain safely and comfortably in your body for several months, provided that careful hygiene measures are used in cleaning and bandaging the catheter site.[6]

Get Someone With Experience!

It takes practice to become skilled at inserting complex central venous catheters. So be sure to ask if the healthcare worker assigned to do your insertion has lots of experience with central lines like yours. If not, ask for someone else.

Q: Once the central venous catheter is in place, could I still develop problems?

A: Central IV lines can become loose and slip out of the vein. Your healthcare worker—and you!—should suspect this if the length of catheter tubing outside your body is getting longer or if you see swelling around the catheter insertion site. That means fluid could be going into your tissues and not into the vein. This should be corrected immediately.[7]

Something else to watch for is possible blocking or kinking of the catheter. Healthcare workers will regularly run clear fluid through your catheter ("flush" it) to keep it clear. If it becomes difficult or impossible to flush, the catheter may be twisted and need repositioning. Total blockage could mean that a blood clot has formed and the catheter may need to be removed and replaced.[7]

Q: These sound like serious problems! And you also said there's a risk of central venous line bloodstream infections. Does this mean I could die from having a central catheter?

A: Central venous catheters are used mostly for critically ill patients in the intensive care unit, who have serious medical conditions that lower their immunity to infection. The risk of central line-related bloodstream infections is also increased for people who need frequent infusions through a central line over a long period of time—for example, people receiving several antibiotics, blood transfusions, parenteral nutrition ("tube feeding"), or kidney dialysis.[9]

So yes, some people do die from infection while a central venous line is in place. Because the catheter is linked directly to the circulation, bacteria that enter the catheter can move throughout the person's entire body, infecting many different organs at the same time. This life-threatening condition is called *septicemia.* Immediate treatment is urgently needed.

Until recently, many other deaths were, in fact, due to central venous line-associated bloodstream infections. But that was *then.* The good news *now* is that hospitals are reducing the risk of these infections, sometimes to *zero,* by following the "bundles" of good clinical practice guidelines I have told you about.[10]

Also realize that most deaths of people who have central line catheters are due to the serious illnesses that made this kind of intensive care treatment necessary. Although there is a risk of infection, the benefit of having a catheter to deliver life-saving drugs and fluids to critically ill patients makes them very valuable for medical care.

I BELIEVE IN ZERO INFECTIONS!

When I was planning this book, several new books were published, that described healthy hospital patients who suddenly developed methicillin-resistant *Staphylococcus aureus* (MRSA) and other incurable infections. These books featured terrible cases of flesh-eating bacteria, limb amputations, and painful, grisly deaths. "Nothing could save them!" many authors wrote.

What good is scaring people about something if you can't do anything to help them? I was determined to show that ordinary people, who had no medical training, could take easy steps to protect themselves from healthcare-associated infections. I had done numerous studies that proved my hand hygiene reminders really worked and helped prevent infections.[11] But I was stymied by the dismal studies reported for central line-associated bloodstream infections.

Careful research had shown that bloodstream infections accounted for 14 percent of all healthcare-associated infections during the 1990s. During that time period, an estimated 250,000 patients developed bloodstream infections in U.S. hospitals every year, and as many as 25 percent of these patients died. In addition to lives lost, the monetary costs for treating these patients averaged approximately $25,000 for each infection.[12] With such dismal findings, could my simple suggestions really help people prevent catheter-related infections?

Now fast-forward to 2002 when the U.S. Centers for Disease Control and Prevention (CDC) issued new guidelines for healthcare workers, designed to help prevent central venous line-associated bloodstream infections.[12] Those guidelines included, among other things, many of the prevention "bundle" measures you just read about:

- Sterile precautions during catheter insertion
- Cleansing the skin with an antiseptic solution before catheter insertion
- Removal of catheters when no longer needed

Researchers at a group of 32 hospitals in southwestern Pennsylvania quickly put these guidelines to the test. First, they collected statistics on the number of central line-associated bloodstream infections that occurred in their intensive care units during 2001. Then, they instituted the new CDC guidelines. By March 2005, just 4 years after using the guidelines, the rate of these bloodstream infections in their medical/surgical intensive care units had decreased by a remarkable *67 percent.*[13]

Based on this proof that central line-associated bloodstream infections can be prevented, the U.S. Centers for Medicare and Medicaid Services (CMS) instituted new regulations in October of 2008, which denied payment to hospitals for certain conditions occurring during a patient's hospital stay that were not present on admission. Central line infections are one of these conditions. What that means is that Medicare and Medicaid will not pay hospitals for the costs of treating these infections if they could have been prevented by good patient care practices.[14] And as you might guess, that's given hospitals tremendous financial incentives to prevent infections.

An added CMS regulation instituted in 2010 now requires hospitals that accept Medicare patients to report all central line-associated bloodstream infections via the CDC's National Healthcare Safety Network (NHSN). These reports are now available to consumers on the government's Hospital Compare website at http://www.hospitalcompare.hhs.gov. Take a look right now to see how well your local hospital is doing to employ infection-prevention measures, compared with other hospitals in your area.[15] These reports have given hospitals even more reasons to stay ahead of their local competitors.

Thanks to required reporting, the first state-by-state infection statistics have already been compiled. During January through June of 2009, more than 1,500 hospitals in 17 states reported an 18 percent decrease in central line-associated bloodstream infections, compared with infection rates that were reported in 2006 through 2008.[16]

That's not as good as the Pennsylvania hospitals' results, and it doesn't come close to some amazing new findings. For example, 90 intensive care units mostly in Michigan (a few in other states) that adopted five infection control guidelines achieved greater than a 60 percent reduction in central catheter-related bloodstream infections at the end of the 36-month study. Many of these hospitals had a zero rate (not even one!) of catheter-related infections during the final 18-month period.[10] A follow-up study showed that patients' risk of dying decreased by about 24 percent in the hospitals that followed these guidelines, compared to only 16 percent decreases in surrounding area hospitals where the program was not in use.[17]

That's why I believe in zero infections! Of course, these findings reflect what's happening at only a small percentage of the over 5,400 hospitals in the United States. Until we can be sure that all hospitals are "at zero," there's more work to be done. Recognizing this, the infection experts at the CDC issued 2011 guidelines, adding even stronger recommendations, such as additional education, training, and knowledge testing for healthcare personnel who treat patients who have IV catheters. The CDC now advises that only trained healthcare workers who have demonstrated their competence should be permitted to insert and maintain peripheral and central intravenous lines.[18]

Other new CDC recommendations include:

- In adults, peripheral IV catheters should be inserted in an upper-extremity (shoulder, arm, forearm, wrist, or hand), rather than a lower extremity (hip, thigh, leg, ankle, or foot).
- Avoid using the femoral vein (in the thigh) for insertion of a central venous catheter.
- At the time a catheter is inserted, the patient should be covered with sterile draping and both the patient and the healthcare worker performing the insertion should wear masks to prevent them from breathing bacteria onto the insertion area.
- Avoid routinely replacing central venous catheters as part of any strategy to prevent infections.

As before, the 2011 CDC guidelines emphasize "bundling" all of the infection control measures together, since skipping even a few recommended practices could outweigh numerous other preventive measures.

YOUR PERSONAL INFECTION-PREVENTION BUNDLE

Even if your hospital has a low infection rate, you still need to be vigilant in reminding your healthcare workers to take precautions when you have a catheter. Hospital workers still need to be reminded to wash their hands before touching a catheter. Bacteria can enter your bloodstream if a catheter is not inserted under sterile conditions. That's the most common way a catheter-associated infection starts.

Catheters can also become contaminated if you have an infection at another area of your body, and the bacteria travel from there to the catheter site. Although it doesn't happen often, solutions used in the catheter bags can get contaminated, too, which means that bacteria can drip directly into your vein.

Be aware that catheter-related bloodstream infections are most likely to occur when a healthcare worker adjusts your catheter:

- During insertion of the catheter
- During dressing changes
- During changing of infusion bags or bottles
- During addition of substances to the infusion bags or bottles

Also keep in mind that a lapse in infection control can be as simple as the healthcare worker's not washing or sanitizing his or her hands before inserting a catheter.

Many hospitals have eliminated these infections, especially by developing hospital infection prevention "bundles" that their healthcare workers must follow. You need a personal central line infection prevention bundle, too! It should include the same five key steps "zero-infection" hospitals are using[10,18-20]:

1. *Hand hygiene:* Hands must be washed before and after contact with a patient.
2. *Barrier precautions:* Sterile technique must be used before, during, and after catheter insertion. This includes wearing a gown, gloves, mask, and cap when inserting the catheter.
3. *Use chlorhexidine skin antiseptics:* The skin should be cleansed with a chlorhexidine solution before the catheter is inserted.
4. *Determine the optimal site for catheter insertion:* Although central venous catheters can be inserted in the subclavian, femoral, or jugular vein, insertion in the subclavian vein is associated with the lowest rate of infection and is the preferred site. The femoral site should be avoided, when possible.

5. *Daily review of the need for a central venous catheter:* Remove the catheter when there is no longer a need for it. The risk of infection increases over time while the catheter remains in place.

Of course, I'm not saying that you should perform all of these procedures by yourself. But I do want you to insist that healthcare workers follow all five of these guidelines, at a minimum.

Similar checklists are used in many of the hospitals that achieved zero infections for patients with central venous catheters.

Central Venous Catheter Checklist

1. *Hand hygiene:* Ask all healthcare workers to wash or sanitize their hands before coming in direct contact with you.
2. *Sterile precautions:* Make sure the person inserting your catheter is wearing a gown, gloves, mask, and cap and is using a sterile pad to prepare the insertion area and that you have full-body drape as well as a mask.
3. *Antibacterial cleansing:* Ask which product will be used to cleanse your skin area before insertion of the catheter. Hospitals should be using chlorhexidine, not iodine. If they aren't using chlorhexidine, *ask that they use it.* All hospitals have this solution readily available.
4. *Catheter removal:* Your need for the catheter should be monitored *each day*. Remember to ask healthcare workers if they have assessed the need for continued catheter insertion.

MARION COSTA LEARNED THAT ONE INFECTION LEADS TO ANOTHER

I have met many victims of healthcare-associated infections through the Consumers Union "Safe Patient Project." The project encourages people to share their difficult stories, which can promote laws to protect patients and provide information to consumers about healthcare quality and safety. That's how I met Marion Costa.

In 2003, 63-year-old Marion was rushed to the hospital for the treatment of an episode of gastrointestinal bleeding. Although it wasn't life-threatening, she needed a transfusion of two pints of blood before being moved to the intensive care unit, After her condition stabilized, she was moved to a regular care unit.

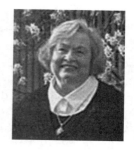

In case she might need additional blood transfusions, the ICU doctors took the precaution of leaving a special catheter (a heparin intravenous lock) in her arm that could be used to deliver the transfused blood. They marked the catheter with a date, ordering it to be removed in three days.

Three days after being admitted to the hospital, Marion experienced a severe headache, backache, and leg pain. She became disoriented and spiked a fever that went up to 105°F. Her doctor administered a powerful sedative to assist in controlling her pain. She awoke 36 hours later, still dangerously ill, but with no memory of what had happened to her.

Results from a blood culture identified her problem: MRSA sepsis—that is, MRSA bacteria in her bloodstream.

Marion was given vancomycin and other antibiotics to treat the infection, but that was just the beginning of her hospital infection ordeal. A week later, her severe gastrointestinal bleeding started again. You may remember from the "superbugs" discussion in Chapter 3 that antibiotic treatment sometimes kills good bacteria along with bad ones like MRSA. That's what had happened to Marion. She developed a second infection from *Clostridium difficile* (*C. diff*) bacteria, because antibiotics had killed the good bacteria that usually prevent *C. diff* from multiplying in the intestinal tract.

Again, Marion required more blood transfusions. However, within a week, she was discharged to a nursing home to continue antibiotic treatment for her MRSA infection. Marion started her advocacy work while in the nursing home. She knew the importance of receiving her antibiotics and when she questioned the nursing staff about receiving them she was told it often takes 3 days after arrival to the nursing home to get the medications.

Did you ever wonder why a doctor will often give you his business card when you are seen in the hospital? Well now Marion knew. It was midnight, she remembered the card that the infectious disease doctor gave her and she called their on-call line. She was immediately seen by a team, antibiotics were ordered and she received them by 2 a.m. Certainly, this was a life-saving tool Marion used and one that I hope you will remember.

You have a right to call either the hospital rapid response line we discussed or your own doctors any time if you believe there is a problem with your care and cannot get results from the staff.

After one week in the nursing home, she again had another high fever, and a few days later, she was transferred by ambulance back to the hospital. She had developed sepsis not with MRSA, but this time with another kind of bacteria that, most likely, had entered her bloodstream through the central venous catheter used to administer her antibiotics. Marion needed treatment with eight different antibiotics to control her bloodstream infection. She considers it as a miracle that she survived this hospital infection nightmare.

Like many patients whose stories you've read in this book, Marion remains angry that her life was endangered by the poor infection control practices that she observed during her hospitalization and nursing home care. For example, while she was in the nursing home, the cap that is used to keep her catheter clean had dropped on the floor and was never found. No one corrected the problem, so she spent a week in the nursing home environment with a dangerously exposed catheter.

After her ordeal, Marion became a tireless advocate for others. Her advocacy work helped to change laws in her state of New Jersey, to improve prevention and reporting of healthcare-associated infections. She continues to work with Consumers Union and the American Association of Retired Persons (AARP) to help others avoid the problems she barely survived.

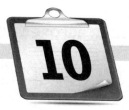

The Challenges of Your
Empowerment Journey

Everything in this book emphasizes two important things:

1. Stay informed and empowered, so that you can protect yourself from infections while you're in the hospital.
2. Wash your hands frequently and insist that healthcare workers do the same.

If you remember just these two things, you are already qualified as a wise consumer of our hospital healthcare system. But consider this: Even if you have a serious illness, you'll spend only a small part of your life as a hospital patient. That's why this guidebook wouldn't be complete without telling you how to prevent infections during the rest of your life. Even when you're not in a hospital, you might be exposed to potentially serious infections that could put you in the hospital.

In addition to being an infection preventionist educator, I'm also a wife, a mother of two children (both now adults), and, until her recent death at age 94, the daughter of an elderly mother. While caring for my loved ones at each stage of their lives, I learned that healthcare empowerment begins even before birth and continues through the last day of life, with many important stops along the way. So, let's begin at birth.

ASK AND TOUR BEFORE YOU DELIVER

You've probably seen the TV commercial showing a pregnant woman and her husband looking at new cars. The announcer says, "You're having a baby, so now you must think about safety when you buy a car." In reality, people spend an average of 8 hours investigating which car to buy, but only 1 hour researching which doctor should perform their surgery.[1]

When a woman is expecting, she'll probably spend lots of time checking out maternity clothes, baby furniture and layettes, or even planning a pre-baby vacation. I hope she'll also spend time to find a highly qualified obstetrician and the best equipped, safest hospital for her baby's delivery.

Tragic Deaths

Early in my career, I was asked to review the tragic death of a newborn who developed an infection because of poor hospital infection control practices. If you knew that your local hospital had this problem, wouldn't you choose to deliver your baby somewhere else? Think about that as you read this real-life example of what happened to several families who chose a poorly run hospital.[2]

Two full-term infants born within 4 days of each other at a small hospital developed sepsis (a severe bloodstream infection) and meningitis (bacterial infection of membranes covering the brain and spinal cord). The cause was found to be an unusual type of *Citrobacter diversus* bacteria. During the investigation, *C. diversus* bacteria were also detected in the rectum or umbilical cord area of 11 out of 40 other infants who were cared for in the nursery during the same time period.

How did such dangerous bacteria get into a newborn nursery? To find out, doctors performed culture tests of tissue samples obtained from two nurses who had been in contact with most of the infected babies shortly after their birth. The cultures from the hands of both nurses and a rectal culture from the second nurse showed the *C. diversus* bacteria. Apparently, the bacteria were carried in by the second nurse, and due to poor hygiene practices in the nursery, *C. diversus* was spread from person to person.

Unfortunately, the problem didn't end there. Six weeks later, continued surveillance at the hospital identified a new group of four newborn infants in the nursery who were infected with the same unusual type of *C. diversus* bacteria. Investigations showed that the mother of one infant was infected with *C. diversus* and had transmitted the infection to her baby during childbirth. Because of poor hygiene in the nursery, the baby's infection spread to other infants.

At this point, the hospital began to use strict infection control procedures, and the outbreak of *C. diversus* infections in the nursery finally ended.

I remember these events very well, because I was asked to help one family to understand what happened to cause the death of their newborn infant. I found several deficiencies in the nursery, but I believe that the most significant problem was their delay in taking appropriate steps to control infections. As a result, infants continued to become infected. The sad part for this family is that they certainly had a choice of other hospitals. Their doctor should have made them aware of that.

Take a Tour

This case occurred over 20 years ago, before the general public knew much about hospital infection risks. But even today, many women simply ask their friends where their babies were delivered, and which doctors they used, or they just choose the most conveniently located obstetrician and hospital. That's not what I recommend. Instead, pregnant women should check on hospital nurseries far in advance of their due date. Here's how to do it:

1. At the time of your first pregnancy visit, ask your obstetrician/gynecologist to obtain infection rate information for the nursery at each hospital you may want to use. Many states have passed laws that require hospitals to collect and report this information. It is your right to see it, so don't be shy about asking. If you are told "Don't worry," I recommend that you find another doctor and another hospital.
2. During your last month of pregnancy, your obstetrician visits will usually switch to a weekly schedule. That's a good time to arrange to tour the nursery at the hospital where you plan to deliver.
3. During the tour, take a note of the following infection control measures:

   - Are the bassinets at least 3 feet apart?
   - Is the nursery overcrowded?
   - Are there enough nurses, or is understaffing a problem?
   - Does the nursery environment look clean and not cluttered?
   - Watch to see whether healthcare workers are washing and sanitizing their hands. Ask how the staff monitors hand hygiene.
   - Ask the nursing supervisor if they've had a cluster or outbreak of infections in the nursery, and how they prevent such infections from spreading.
   - Ask whether the hospital's infection control division is currently investigating any infection incidents in the nursery.

Nursery Checklist

1. Obtain infection rate statistics for the nursery at each hospital you may want to use.
2. At the start of your last month of pregnancy, tour each nursery and observe whether healthcare workers are washing and sanitizing their hands, and whether other infection control measures are being used.
3. Ask the nursing supervisor whether outbreaks of infection have occurred in the nursery and whether any infection control investigations are in progress.
4. If you aren't satisfied with the conditions in the nursery, even this late in your pregnancy, take time to find another hospital. Your baby's life could depend on it!

HOW TO FIND A SAFE DAY CARE

If you've ever had a baby, I hope you asked all the right questions and were pleased with the hospital care you and your baby received. But a mother's work is never done, as they say. For many parents who work outside the home, the next milestone is searching for the perfect day care center.

I've been there, done that. As a budding new professor at an Ivy League University when I had our first child, I knew I needed to find day care. I hope you can learn from my experience.

How did I handle the situation? Using my research skills, I designed a hands-on study to investigate conditions at day care centers I would consider for our son. I obtained agreements from 12 licensed centers in urban Philadelphia to observe their infection control practices (graduate students assisted in this) and then provide in-service education to instruct their workers about proper hygiene measures.[3]

What Did We Find?

We scheduled our visits at different times of the day so we could observe the full range of activities. At one center, we saw food preparation taking place in the same area used for changing diapers, with nothing used to cover the diapering area. In some centers, cribs were packed so close together that workers couldn't walk between them. Toys used at every center were frequently contaminated with "body secretions" from sneezing and drooling children, but they were not cleaned regularly. All staff members said they washed their hands after using the bathroom, but only 82 percent did so after diaper changing, and only 27 percent washed their hands between contacts with sick and well children.

Good Times, Bad Times

As if these problems weren't enough, the observation that concerned me most was the difference we saw during the day versus drop-off and pick-up times. For example, when children were dropped off or picked up, the centers were always well-organized and children were cared for. However, when we went to the center to collect our data during the day, it seemed like total chaos, with kids crying and roaming around. This was not the well-organized appearance that the centers presented when parents were there to observe.

As mothers know, days with a young toddler can be very stressful. Just multiply that by 20 or 30 stressed-out toddlers, and you can see that the demand can be overwhelming. Also, we realized that day care center workers are often paid minimum salaries and that might affect their performance.

Our study was published in a prominent medical journal, bringing considerable attention to my healthcare concerns. Since then, I am glad to say, there has been a great deal of improvement in day care. One reason is that centers began to employ infection control consultants from their local communities to assist in developing policies and practices to prevent the transmission of disease.

Take It Along

One notable consultant, an Iowa nurse-epidemiologist, Peggy Christ, RN, ET, CIC, created and publicized *The Ten Infection Control Commandments of Child Day Care*, which provided guidelines for infection control in day care centers around the country.[4] Her list of "You shall" commandments includes:

You shall . . .

- Follow procedures to prevent the spread of contagious diseases *always*, not just when a child in the center is already ill.
- Wash and disinfect toilets, faucet handles, and other bathroom surfaces more than once a day, if possible.
- Use washable toys, especially with diapered children.

- Be sure caregivers of diapered children do not *prepare* food and do not *serve* food to children outside their own group of children.
- Enforce all immunization requirements.
- Perform hand-washing as the most important action that children and staff do to prevent the spread of infection.

Although the list was developed for day care workers, it is a good document to take along on your tour of day care centers for your children.

KIDS—AND GERMS—GO TO SCHOOL

When a child ages out of day care or home care, it's time for that emotional first day at school. Like hospitals, schools are a major source of infection for children. Why? First of all, children in school are grouped very close to one another, and they share many objects such as toys, pencils, books, computers, and more, all of which can pass bacteria and viruses from one child to another. That is, if children do not practice good hand hygiene.

Communicable infections such as colds, flu, and stomach viruses are a major cause of school absenteeism.[5] The most recent national survey of U.S. children aged 5–17 years showed that 4 percent of all children missed 11 or more days of school due to illness or injury during the year 2007. Almost 15 percent of all children missed 6 or more days of school during that year.[6] In another study, researchers found that about 25 percent of elementary students in San Diego County (California) were absent at least 5 percent of the time during the 2008–2009 school year. As in the national study, poor and minority children had higher rates of absenteeism, often due to lack of healthcare.[7]

We know that handwashing could help to prevent infections, but can it reduce absenteeism in schools? In 2002, we did a follow-up study in which we created a hand-washing education program that five independent schools presented in their health classes.[8]

We called it the "Buddies Handwashing Program," because "Buddies watch out for one another." The program required only 1 hour of instruction time and was very easy to implement:

1. Every classroom had a dispenser of sanitizer placed on the wall.
2. Kids listened to a lecture about bacteria and were shown how to wash their hands correctly.
3. They were told that they need to use the sanitizer if they sneezed, after using the bathroom, and before and after eating lunch.
4. They completed a word search game that contained handwashing terms such as soap, towel, water, and bathroom.

5. As a final test, all the children demonstrated to the teacher how they sanitized their hands.

The reward was a colorful "Healthy Hands, Healthy Kids" card to carry in their wallet, which said they were "Ambassadors of Good Health."

Cost Savings, Too

We were pleased to find that absenteeism was 50 percent lower in the test classrooms where students were taught to use sanitizer. In terms of teachers' time for remedial work and other costs, we calculated that schools saved an average of $167.00 for each student who participated in the program.

The lesson for parents is to keep reminding your children to wash and sanitize their hands throughout their day at school and also at home.

GERMS AT WORK IN YOUR OFFICE

Adults should be careful about hand hygiene, too, especially at work. That's because germs cause illness, and illness results in absenteeism, which is costly for employees and businesses. For example, statistics in the United Kingdom for 2009 through 2010 showed that over 28 million work days were lost overall that year (1.2 days per worker), of which over 23 million were due to work-related ill health.[9]

Unclean Hands

During the 1990s, when worldwide outbreaks of swine flu were feared, health officials recognized that flu germs would be transmitted via people's unclean hands. Therefore, they recommended installation of sanitizer dispensers in public places and office buildings. The public responded positively, but when the flu alert ended, sanitizer use decreased. Nevertheless, infection control experts wondered if continued promotion of sanitizers in the workplace would lead to fewer lost work days.

Research currently points in that direction. In one recent study, German researchers divided a large public administration building into two sections; hand sanitizers were installed in one section, but not in the other section. The result was that people in the hand sanitizer section had fewer episodes of common colds, fever, and coughing, and they took fewer days off from work.[10]

Does your workplace have sanitizer dispensers installed in office areas? What about in restrooms? If not, tell your boss that those dispensers could save the company lots of money in lost work days. Of course, sanitizers won't do much good if you don't use them. You have to play an active role in protecting yourself from infections.

Germs on the Menu

Do you eat lunch or snacks at your office desk? Well, here's some information that could change your mind. According to a study by a University of Arizona microbiologist who collected bacteria samples in offices around the country, your office desk probably harbors 400 times more bacteria than your office bathroom toilet seat! Even a small area on your desk or phone can host over 10 million bacteria that could make you sick.[11]

The study also showed that surfaces in personal work spaces such as offices or cubicles actually have higher bacteria levels than surfaces in common areas. For example, here's what researchers found in 7,000 bacterial samples collected from typical offices, cubicles, and open work spaces in New York City, San Francisco, Tampa (Florida), and Tucson (Arizona):

- Phone receivers: average 25,127 bacteria per square inch
- Desktop: average 20,961 bacteria per square inch
- Computer keyboard: average 3,295 bacteria per square inch
- Computer mouse: average 1,676 bacteria per square inch

When office workers were instructed to use alcohol-based disinfectant wiping cloths (from Clorox, the study sponsor) to clean their desks after lunch, bacteria levels were reduced by 99 percent or more. The moral of the story: If you still want to keep eating at your desk, remember to clean it before and after.

HOW SAFE ARE AMBULATORY SURGERY CENTERS?

Years ago, people who needed surgery usually remained in the hospital for several days, weeks, or even months, until they and their doctor felt it was safe to go home. Today, that's just a distant memory, as high medical costs and insurance company restrictions permit only short hospital stays or even no hospital admission at all for many surgical procedures.

If you need minor surgery or an invasive test (colonoscopy, for example), chances are that you'll be sent to an ambulatory surgery center. Expect to arrive in the morning and be back home in the evening, even if you feel you need more nursing care and observation.

Dirty Secrets

Ambulatory surgery centers are not hospitals. Although they look very similar, the emphasis here is on moving patients in and out quickly. It's natural to worry that details like infection control measures could be overlooked, but there's less need to worry these days. As we often say about healthcare-associated infections, "the dirty secrets are out" and healthcare facilities are being more careful.

More than 5,000 ambulatory care centers in the United States participate in the Medicare program. So it should reassure you to know that as of January 2010, Medicare regulations now require its member centers to follow infection control guidelines.[12]

Patients still need to be on their guard because the guidelines don't include specific steps that must be taken at every facility. In fact, the standards are so loose that ambulatory care facilities are free to establish their own infection control programs.

Frequent "Lapses"

How is this working out? Not very well, according to recent inspections conducted by the U.S. Centers for Disease Control and Prevention and the Centers for Medicaid Services at 68 ambulatory surgery centers in Maryland, North Carolina, and Oklahoma.[13] Infection control "lapses" were found at more than two out of three of these facilities. Almost 18 percent of the centers did poorly on three or more of the five categories of infection control that were investigated.

The most common infection risks involved reuse of blood glucose testing equipment meant for only a single use and use of single-dose medication vials for more than one patient. Overall, 57 percent of the centers were given "citations" because of deficiencies in infection control.

Hard to believe, but these failures occurred when healthcare workers knew that they were being watched. Who knows how many more infection control lapses occur when no inspectors are present? Also remember that many ambulatory surgery centers are not accredited by Medicare and aren't regularly inspected.

An editorial accompanying the report about infection control lapses noted that more than 6 million patients each year undergo procedures at ambulatory surgery centers, which means that several million patients could face the risk of healthcare-associated infections. According to the author, "This risk is not acceptable and must be corrected immediately and definitely."

Consider the Advantages

That's the bad news. The good news is that infection control lapses don't always mean that patients will develop infections. Also, many people welcome the lower cost of out-of-hospital surgery, tests, and treatment, and the ability to go back home the same day. Some believe that infection risks are greater at hospitals filled with seriously ill patients.

Whether this is your preference or not, it's definitely the wave of the present and the future. The Ambulatory Surgery Center Association estimates that since 1970 when the first center opened, the number of centers has increased from 2,786 in 1999 to 4,506 in 2005, with growth continuing at over 8 percent each a year.[14]

TIPS FOR SAFE RECOVERY AT HOME

Whether you've had surgery, tests, and treatments in a hospital or at an ambulatory care center, your greatest risk of infection problems could actually be when you're back at home. That's because you're on your own to change bandages, check for healing problems, fill your own prescriptions, prepare meals, and perform your usual activities without skilled help. Unless you've had professional training, you may not have the knowledge to perform needed care procedures or to know when you absolutely must get immediate medical help.

In addition, healthcare-associated infections often take a week or more to cause symptoms, so problems may not be evident at the time you're sent home after surgery. That's what happened to a woman I'll call "Mrs. N," whose same-day surgery turned into 16 months of complications.

When Mrs. N was 67 years old, she complained about knee problems. Her doctor recommended performing an arthroscopic examination of the affected knee. The procedure involves inserting a tiny viewing scope through a small incision in the knee, so a surgeon can look inside, locate, and remove scar tissue that is causing pain and stiffness. This "debridement" procedure is relatively safe, so it is often done at a same-day (ambulatory) surgery center.

Although Mrs. N had diabetes, it was well controlled with oral medications and her overall health was good. Her diabetes wasn't thought to be a problem that would necessitate in-hospital surgery. Mrs. N arrived at the surgery center early in the morning, had the procedure, and went home the same day. However, 15 days later, her knee continued to be very painful. She needed to go back for another arthroscopy and debridement. Cultures of fluid from her knee revealed a serious *Staphylococcus aureus* infection.

At that point, Mrs. N's family decided to have her transferred to a larger medical center, where she underwent a third operation, this time with a surgical open incision. Again, cultures of fluid in her knee showed *Staph aureus*. As a result, Mrs. N had to spend a week in the hospital for intravenous administration of antibiotics, followed by a full month of care at a rehabilitation facility. It was a long 16 months after her first surgery when she was told her infection was finally gone. The surgeon said that she could now have knee replacement surgery to relieve her persistent pain, but she refused to take the risk of another operation.

Consider the Evidence

I met Mrs. N when she decided to file a lawsuit against the ambulatory surgery center and take the matter to court. I was asked to be an expert witness for this case. My role was to review her records to determine whether the ambulatory surgery center had put Mrs. N at risk for the infection. What I found was surprising:

1. Patients treated by the surgeon who performed her procedure at the center had a record of more infections than occurred with other surgeons doing the same type of procedure.
2. In the year of Mrs. N's surgery, the surgery center had a 20 percent increase in *Staph aureus* infections.
3. During that year, the surgery center reported six infections that occurred after this type of surgery, five of which were *Staph aureus* infections.
4. All five patients with *Staph aureus* had been treated by the same surgeon as Mrs. N.

With all this evidence, I am sure you are thinking, "Wow! Mrs. N must have gotten a good verdict and lots of money." Actually, she lost the case. Why? Well, the opposing attorney was able to convince the jury that Mrs. N's diabetes was the cause of her infections, because diabetics have a greater risk for infections.

The defense attorney also pointed out that the surgeon had diagnosed the infection and treated it, which doesn't provide any proof that the surgeon caused the infection. The jury focused on these statements and not on the fact that Mrs. N's well-controlled diabetes did not increase her risk for an infection. It didn't seem to matter to the jury that other patients treated by Mrs. N's surgeon also developed the same *Staph aureus* infections.

If Only She Had Known

Throughout the book, I've emphasized how important it is to check infection statistics for any health facility before you decide to be treated there. If only Mrs. N had known about infection problems at the ambulatory care center, she could have chosen a different facility. She told me that she preferred some place closer to her home, but isn't it better to be further away and without risk of surgical complications?

So what could Mrs. N have done to stay safe, apart from not choosing a facility known to have infection troubles? Here's what healthcare experts advise for every patient treated at ambulatory surgery facilities[15]:

1. Be sure the facility is affiliated with a hospital. If it is not, ask in advance how the staff will handle an emergency that might occur during your procedure.
2. Bring a list of the medicines, dietary supplements, and over-the-counter medications you take, and mention any drugs you're allergic to, so the staff will know which medications may be needed during the time you are there.
3. Before your procedure, if you have diabetes like Mrs. N, remind the staff to monitor your glucose level before, during, and after surgery.
4. When you are being discharged to go home, ask about potential complications from your surgery that you should look for, whom to call if problems arise, what days you have been scheduled for follow-up appointments, and whether you will receive a follow-up phone call from the ambulatory facility to check on your recovery. (Studies show that follow-up calls help to prevent complications and readmissions to care facilities.[16])
5. If you are given prescriptions to fill, ask for a written list and a full explanation so that you can understand what the medicines are, when you're supposed to take them, and how long you'll need them. If there's something you don't understand, ask for it to be explained in simple language.
6. If you're given equipment to use—for example, crutches, a walker, cane, urinary catheter, or oxygen mask, to name but a few—be sure you get a full demonstration of how to use it and then demonstrate how you can do it yourself.
7. If you are concerned or unclear about something that is being explained or done to you, speak up and ask questions. Bring an advocate who can speak for you if you're too disabled or weak to do so.

8. Visit your primary care doctor soon after you get home, because that doctor is now responsible for your follow-up care and can spot problems before they become serious.[17]

Ambulatory Care Checklist

You need to be an empowered patient to stay safe during and after treatment at an ambulatory surgery center. Ask questions and don't hesitate to speak up if you are concerned or unclear about something that healthcare workers are doing.

1. Bring an advocate with you who can speak for you if you're unable to do so.
2. Before your surgery or treatment, remind the staff of any medications you're taking that you may need during your stay.
3. When you're discharged to go home, ask about symptoms to watch for, whom to call if problems arise, and when you're scheduled for a follow-up appointment.
4. Get a full explanation about any prescriptions and equipment that you will need to use at home.
5. See your primary doctor for follow-up care soon after you get home.

FACING THE HEALTH CHALLENGES OF GROWING OLDER

Most people do make a good recovery after outpatient treatments, but elderly people often need more time, and help, to recover. Fortunately, there are many options for continued care of the elderly. Unfortunately, making the right choice can be difficult, especially because it could determine the course of the rest of the patient's life.

The best way to start is to evaluate the following three main factors[18]:

1. *The patient's personal goals,* such as getting rehabilitation to return to independent living, or finding a safer living situation, or obtaining continued medical supervision.

2. *Family circumstances and resources*, such as having the time and ability to help with the patient's continued care at home, available insurance coverage for care outside the home, or financial ability to pay for at-home or outside care.

3. *The patient's health history*, which may determine whether continued medical care might improve his or her functioning or prevent further deterioration.

Finding the Best Service or Facility

The final step is choosing a service or care facility. In the same way you would evaluate a hospital, an ambulatory care facility, a newborn nursery, or a day care center, you'll certainly want to tour several facilities before making a choice. Check for cleanliness, hygiene practices, and the activities you see during your tour. Be sure to talk to residents. Of course, you'll inquire about the facility's accreditation and inspection history.

Location is always a factor, but don't make it the main factor. Although many families choose the closest facility so that visiting is easier, it's better to travel a bit farther rather than jeopardize the patient's health and safety at a nonaccredited center.

There's much more you'll need to know if you're choosing a care center. I've listed many helpful sources of information in the Resources section at the end of the book, but for a quick start, check out:

- *For assisted living facilities:* The Assisted Living Federation of America's "Guide to Choosing an Assisted Living Community." http://www.alfa. org/images/alfa/PDFs/PublicationsResources/Guide_to_Choosing_ Assisted_Living_Community.pdf.

- *For nursing homes:* The Centers for Medicare & Medicaid Services online quality report "Nursing Home Compare." http://www.medicare. gov/NHCompare/Include/DataSection/Questions/SearchCriteriaNEW. asp and "Navigating the Healthcare System: Tools to Help you Choose a Good Nursing Home" by Carolyn M. Claney, M.D. http://www.ahrq. gov/consumer/cc/cc/20611.htm

IS ASSISTED LIVING YOUR BEST CHOICE?

In the United States, most people who need continuing care that can't be provided at home will move to an assisted living facility or a nursing home. That's why I'll focus on these two choices.

Do you know anyone who has an apartment in an assisted living community? You probably do, because about 1 million people in the United States currently reside in assisted living facilities. That number is projected to double by 2030.[19] Federal regulations define an assisted living facility as an institutional setting that "provides managed delivery of health and personal care services within a residential environment." Most residents live in their own rooms, but can call on staff members for assistance.[20,21]

Are They Regulated?

Assisted living facilities are not subject to federal government regulation. Although all 50 states license or "certify" these facilities, the states currently provide very little regulation and oversight.[20,22]

You just read that recent inspections found serious infection control lapses at more than two-thirds of ambulatory care facilities. Can you imagine how many more lapses may be occurring at any kind of care facility that doesn't face inspections? There's no need to imagine, because many infection problems have indeed been reported at assisted living facilities.

In 2005, for example, two outbreaks of hepatitis B virus infection occurred at assisted living facilities in Virginia. Infections were traced to multiple use of finger-stick devices that are meant for only a single use to obtain a blood sample for glucose testing in diabetic patients. Concerned by these findings, the Virginia Department of Social Services and the Centers for Disease Control sent education materials to assisted living facilities throughout Virginia to inform them of the proper methods for infection control and glucose monitoring.[21]

During a later survey of 55 facilities, inspectors found that 20 percent of facilities were still sharing finger-stick devices between residents. Many facilities were deficient in sterile glove usage, and one-third of the facilities did not have a sink near medication areas and nursing stations for the staff to wash their hands. Overall, more than one out of every three assisted living facilities that were surveyed was found to be noncompliant with federal infection control guidelines.[21]

These lapses aren't confined to Virginia. For example, similar hepatitis B virus outbreaks have been reported in North Carolina.[23] In Arizona, recent investigations revealed frequent lack of supervision by professional nurses in assisted living facilities where unlicensed personnel were administering complex medications, and staff members had been accused of physical, verbal, psychological, and sexual abuse.[24]

What I Observed

The problem with many assisted living facilities is that they want to present a home-like atmosphere. They give less thought to the infection control practices needed for people who are living in such close contact and who require basic healthcare procedures such as finger sticks. I knew that these facilities are not required to follow specific infection control guidelines, so I did some research to see what they actually were doing. Here's the unconvincing assurance I found posted at many facilities:

> *Each facility must establish and maintain an infection control policy and procedure designated to provide a safe, sanitary, and comfortable environment and to help prevent the development and transmission of disease and infection.*

FROM ASSISTED LIVING, BACK TO HOME

I know what to look for in healthcare facilities. I have extensive experience investigating complaints about medical care. I know that some assisted living facilities don't come close to meeting recognized care standards. When I needed to find a good facility for my mother, I sadly learned that even my extensive knowledge didn't make the task any easier . . . or the result any better.

My mother, Anna McGuckin, had been living independently in her own two-story home. At age 94, she had no medical issues other than short-term memory deficits. In fact, she had never been in the hospital. Still, my daughter and I worried about her safety, so we began to investigate assisted living facilities. I believed that at age 94, that kind of facility would be a safer choice for her than remaining at home. She'd have some daily companionship and there wouldn't be any steps to climb. My daughter offered to accompany me to these facilities because this can be a very emotional decision.

First Meeting

At each of the 10 facilities we visited, we saw what we called "the white carpeted executive suite" where visitors were greeted. There was nice furniture, happy staff members, and "simply by chance," an introduction to someone who had just moved a relative into the facility and "knew how we were feeling."

Rule 1: Don't be fooled by a first meeting. Take time to ask if patients actually get to use this luxurious part of the facility!

Rule 2: Don't think your wishes will be followed. In these facilities, healthcare workers often assume that a person who is a little confused must have a urinary tract infection, even if, as was my Mom's case, she has no symptoms. I agreed to have her give a urine specimen in a cup for testing, but I made certain to put a note in her chart that no catheterization should be done to obtain a specimen. Despite that, they did a catheterization, and of course, found no urinary infection.

Rule 3: Check for infection control. During my Mom's short stay, I saw many basic infection control practices not being followed. For me, the worst offense was lack of easy access to sanitizers and obvious non-compliance with handwashing guidelines.

Rule 4: Report and speak out. Although I definitely planned to file a complaint about the facility, I first made my complaints known to the director, thinking my input would help the staff and the residents. Did it help? Their response was a letter to me saying they did not believe their facility was "a good fit" for my Mom. More likely, they felt my careful scrutiny was too risky for their comfort. So Mom went back to her home and with a little help, returned to her old self.

Yes, I did follow-up by calling our state and county health departments. I must say, if you are in this situation, DO IT! It is easy to do, but just be sure you document your concerns by giving specific examples of what went wrong. In my case, health inspectors actually went to the assisted care facility on a Sunday morning, clearly taking them by surprise, and asked that the Director be called. The authorities followed up with me on what they discovered, and what the facility needed to do to comply with their findings.

Rule 5: Surprise is an important tactic, as I just mentioned. When I was visiting facilities for my Mom, a colleague of mine shared an observation based on her many years of doing physical therapy work in assisted living facilities. She said staff members learn very quickly when residents' families usually visit. That way, they make absolutely certain to have the resident bathed and in good shape before family members are due to arrive. Need I say more?

Visit and Inspect

Many assisted living facilities prominently post a list of residents' rights, but the real issue is how to make these facilities safe 24/7. Although they now have no specific guidelines or regulatory demands, many excellent assisted living centers do care about their residents' health, safety, and enjoyment. Moreover, most residents enjoy the lifestyle, companionship, recreational activities, and needed help that assisted living offers.

Local, state, and federal agencies are now performing more monitoring and inspection visits, so don't give up on assisted living facilities. Just be very diligent about visiting and inspecting before—and after—you choose a facility for yourself or a family member. Our elderly family members, like our children, are extremely vulnerable. They need our advocacy.

My Mom died in July 2010 in her own home. I shared her story here because she was an inspiration throughout my career. Even at 94, she helped me do for others by taking action to report problems at her assisted living facility (although she didn't realize I had done so). It would have been easier for me to say, "Not my problem," but the faces of many elderly people in this facility made it too hard not to speak out.

NURSING HOMES AND OTHER LONG-TERM CARE FACILITIES

People with serious chronic, incurable illnesses are not permitted to remain in the hospital as long as used to be the practice, but assisted living facilities aren't equipped to meet their needs. These days, *long-term care facilities* take over where the hospitals leave off. According to March 2011 statistics, about 1.4 million people are currently residing in a total of 15,000 U.S. long-term care facilities.[25]

What Is a Nursing Home?

By definition, long-term care facilities are institutions that provide health-care to people who are unable to manage independently in the community.[20] Nursing homes are a special category of long-term care facilities that provide inpatient beds and an organized professional staff who supply continuous nursing care and other services to patients who have chronic illnesses.[26]

Finding a Good Nursing Home

If a loved one needs nursing home care, a good way to start your search is by asking your doctor, hospital discharge planner, or community social service agency to recommend several nursing homes in the area you're focusing on.

You should know that all long-term care facilities, including nursing homes, are required by law to follow the same infection control guidelines that hospitals must follow.[26] Be very skeptical if a facility director tells you that their nursing home uses different guidelines. Although it may sound funny, bacteria don't know the difference between hospitals and nursing homes.

The Joint Commission, which I've mentioned before, is a good starting point to help you find a good nursing home. The Commission collects information about the safety and quality of every care organization that receives Joint Commission Accreditation. Each of these facilities undergoes an on-site survey every 3 years, so you'll have some assurance of good care if you choose an accredited nursing home.

Check the Commission's website to find accredited nursing homes in your search area (www.jointcommission.org). Then go to the Commission's Quality Check® website (www.qualitycheck.org) to see detailed information about each nursing home's performance and how the facility compares to similar institutions.

See for Yourself

Looking at a website is no substitute for being there yourself, so make sure to visit each nursing home, take a tour, and talk with the manager or other staff members about the organization's services, policies, history, and staff credentials.

Nursing Home Checklist

■ Does the building look and smell clean and well cared for?

■ Are sinks and sanitizers easy to access throughout the building to ensure good hand hygiene by residents, healthcare workers, and visitors?

■ Are many staff members present, or is the facility "short staffed"?

- How many registered nurses are on the staff? (Studies indicate this is a strong predictor of quality care.)

- Can you speak with several residents and their families in private, where they won't worry that negative comments may be overheard by the staff?

Infection Risks

The director at each nursing home should tell you what the facility is doing to prevent and manage infection risks. That's one of the most important facts you should know when you're choosing a nursing home. Here's why: Many patients these days are discharged quickly from acute care settings, often before healthcare-associated infections have started to cause symptoms. So the infections people bring into long-term care facilities are very similar to those in acute care hospitals.[26]

In addition, chronically ill and frail elderly people who need nursing home care often have decreased resistance to infections. Consequently, the infection rate in long-term care facilities is equal to or higher than acute care hospitals.[27]

The risk of rapidly spreading infection outbreaks is especially high in nursing homes because residents live together in a confined space where they share the same air, food, water, and healthcare providers.[28] Outbreaks of influenza and other respiratory tract infections are especially common and easily spread in the nursing home environment.[29] In fact, U.S. statistics show that between 1.6 and 3.8 million outbreaks of infection occur each year in long-term care facilities, with associated costs exceeding 1 billion dollars.[27]

Protection for Residents

To protect residents and staff, nursing homes that accept Medicare and Medicaid reimbursement are required to have:

"A comprehensive infection control program designed to provide a safe, sanitary, and comfortable environment, and to help prevent the development and transmission of disease and infection."[26]

The infection control program should follow recommended care guidelines, including:

- Surveillance of infections
- Management of infection outbreaks

- Risk assessment
- Isolation measures
- Monitoring of antibiotic use
- Hand hygiene practices
- Standards for processing and storage of linens
- Staff safety

All nursing homes and other long-term care facilities are also required to offer each resident and staff member immunization against influenza and lifetime immunization against pneumococcal disease (pneumonia).[26]

IMPROVING THE SYSTEM

As an infection preventionist, I could not sit back and do nothing about preventing infections in nursing homes. So in 2002, my colleagues and I developed a program to educate long-term care workers about basic hand hygiene practices.[30]

We began the program at three large long-term care centers by asking staff members what they actually knew about hand hygiene. Only 28 percent of the workers knew when they should wash their hands, and only 3 percent knew why it was important to wash their hands after removing protective gloves.

We found that the healthcare workers were very open to making improvements, but just didn't know proper hygiene practices. We educated them with videos, posters, lectures, and demonstrations during a 6- to 8-week period. Raffle prizes were awarded at each education session to maintain interest. When the workers learned what to do, they improved significantly. For example, after the program, proper handwashing and sanitizer use increased by an overall 52 percent. In some centers, infection rates also decreased.

During the 8 weeks of our study, we saw a constant turnover of staff. That means nursing home workers need frequent reminders about care guidelines, so that the information reaches even the newest staff members.

Make the System Work!

I've shared the stories and research studies in this chapter so you can see how important it is for you to be an empowered caregiver for yourself and those you love. Empowerment is necessary to change our current medical care away from a big business system that focuses on operations and finances to one that instead focuses attention on meeting each patient's care needs.

When it comes to long-term care, all I can say is that our society tolerates the current care system because we believe this is what our elderly want. Granted, for some who need skilled nursing care, options are very few. But there is no reason why we can't make our entire long-term care system work better.

I hope that after reading this chapter, you can see that empowerment needs to be a part of every stage of life. Taking just few simple steps to protect yourself and your loved ones that can make a big difference in preventing illness and disability.

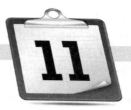

Calling in the Law, or Not

In medicine, choices that doctors make can mean the difference between life and death or improved health and permanent disability. Physicians are guided by the Hippocratic Oath to "Do no harm," but mistakes are sometimes made. When a physician fails to fulfill a duty owed to the patient and injury results, there are certainly consequences, sometimes including lawsuits. However, people have different opinions about the act of suing a hospital or a physician, from those who feel such claims lack merit, to those who support a patient's right to recover any damages and punish the wrongdoer.

A longtime friend of mine is a practicing plaintiff attorney, which means his clients (the plaintiffs) are patients who have been harmed by our healthcare system. Here's what he once shared with me and my students during his guest lecture in my University of Pennsylvania class on Adverse Events in Healthcare:

> In all my years as a plaintiff attorney, I can tell you there is one thing that I can guarantee 100%, and that is I have never had a happy client. I find that if my client wins, the money does not bring back a person or remove the suffering. If I lose a case, my clients continue to be angry.

I hesitated on whether to include this chapter about lawsuits—or, more correctly, malpractice claims—because, up to this point, I have tried just to teach you the steps to prevent infections. However, there will always be infections. Therefore, it is important for you to know what legal steps you may want or need to take, and how to justify your decision. Since this chapter is titled *Calling in the Law, or Not*, I want the information to help you understand not just your options, but also the consequences of each option.

As you can imagine, it is hard to find a lawyer who will share "just the facts," as I like to say. However, I do have the perfect person to do this. Do you remember that budding middle-school researcher who observed fellow students not washing their hands I wrote about earlier? Well, Maryellen Guinan is now an attorney who concentrates on health law. Why would she not do this chapter for her mother?

Think Before You Sue

By Maryellen E. Guinan, Esquire

In 2005, my older brother John, at the time a junior at University of Pennsylvania, conducted a study of Pennsylvania malpractice claims related to healthcare-associated infections. He found that the highest number of cases occurred in the specialties of orthopedics, general surgery, and cardiothoracic medicine (related to the heart and other organs in the chest).[1] The sites infected most often were the knees, back, sternum (breast bone), and harvest sites (leg or chest areas from which a vein or artery is removed for use in coronary artery bypass surgery and other procedures).

Of the 154 cases included in John's published study, 27 were withdrawn, 27 settled without a trial, 11 still pending, 9 won by the plaintiff (the injured person), and 5 won by the defense (the doctor or hospital).[1] Despite his finding that 72 percent of these Philadelphia malpractice cases were either withdrawn or settled, John found that it was advantageous to go to trial, since 60 percent of those who did so won their cases. By the way, John became an attorney.

LAWSUITS: THE GOOD, THE BAD, AND THE UGLY

The cost of medical malpractice in the United States is $55.6 billion a year, which is 2.4 percent of annual healthcare spending.[2] That's a lot of money, but don't assume you'll get a lot of money by suing. The amount you might receive isn't always proportional to the amount of negligence you may have suffered.

First, it's important to realize there's a probability that the case will be settled without ever seeing the inside of a courtroom. Second, be aware that if the case does go to trial, it's still a gamble as to how the jury will decide and what the award could be. Juries vary from state to state and from case to case; therefore, it is nearly impossible to predict the outcome for any particular trial.

How big a gamble is it? Just think about Mrs. N, the woman with the terrible knee infection whose case you read about earlier. I am certain she never thought about alternatives to calling in the law. She believed harm had been done to her by a surgeon with a bad record, and she was sure that the jury would see it that way, too. She never imagined how defense lawyers could turn the case around, making everything seem like her fault. She also didn't realize that in the small town where her case was tried, there was a good chance that several jurors would know the doctor and the hospital.

Legal Fees

What other shortcomings and unintended effects should you think about before deciding to sue? Most importantly, don't count on full compensation. Administrative costs for legal and processing fees will probably eat up more than 50 percent of any money you're awarded.[3]

Also, don't assume that lawyers will want to take your case, even if your claim has merit. Unfortunately, lesser claims (those not yielding a large cash verdict) may not be attractive because the costs of proving that malpractice has occurred are likely to exceed the award. In contrast, claims lacking great merit are often brought to trial because lawyers believe the plaintiff is so "sympathetic" (a child with permanent injuries who will not be able to attend college or have a career, for instance) that they are likely to receive a windfall from a generous jury.

High and Low

Furthermore, don't be deceived by huge monetary awards that are publicized in newspapers and other mainstream media. Behind the big dollar numbers is the reality that plaintiffs often settle for less than the jury awards. Here's how it happens: Before a verdict comes in, for example, while a jury is deliberating, both sides may sign a "high-low agreement" that guarantees that the victim will receive at least some minimum amount of money (the "low"), but not more than a capped amount (the "high"). Thus, a seemingly high jury award may be capped at a lesser amount via these agreements.[4]

Damages

What, then, is the "proper amount" of compensation, and what form should it take? The law recognizes three categories of recoverable "damages" in cases involving wrongful action that causes harm (a "tort action"): (1) compensatory, (2) punitive, and (3) nominal.[5]

> *Compensatory damages*, in the medical liability context, place a monetary value on the injuries incurred by the patient and the costs of future medical care that is needed as a result of the medical error or negligence. The overall "cost" of an injury is not limited to the patient's hospital bills, but also includes nursing services, physical therapy, drug costs, lost wages, and diminished earning capacity of the injured person, among other expenses. Your lawyer may call on medical experts to testify about your future medical needs, and also an economist to estimate future expenses based on your life expectancy, inflation, and other factors.[5]

> *Punitive damages* are awarded to punish the defendant (the healthcare provider and/or hospital) to potentially deter others from the same bad behavior or to gain justice for you, the plaintiff. The jury must find that the defendant acted in such a repulsive manner based on clear and convincing evidence.[6]

> *Nominal damages*, the final category, represent an award given to the plaintiff to show a legal wrong was committed and the plaintiff suffered as a result, but did not have sufficient or actual damage that would require compensation. The nominal award (usually one dollar), is the court's way of acknowledging that a legal wrongdoing has occurred.[6]

If you were the plaintiff, would you be satisfied with nominal damages? After a long and costly lawsuit, probably not. But that could be all you'll come away with.

APOLOGY: IS "I'M SORRY" ENOUGH?

Even if you do receive a nice settlement, you may not feel satisfied because there's no mechanism within the courts to guarantee that corrective action will be taken, or that you'll receive an apology, or even an expression of regret and concern. So, it's important for you to ask yourself, "What is my true goal in suing? To gain money or is it something else?"

Extra-Legal Rewards

It really doesn't have to be about money. "Extra-legal" (non-monetary) objectives often motivate people to sue for medical malpractice.[7] More than dollars, you may be eager for:

- Apologies and admissions of fault
- Receiving retribution for the doctor's conduct (a public reprimand, perhaps)
- Obtaining answers to what had gone wrong in your treatment
- Having steps taken to prevent recurrences

Assuming you are sure of what you really want, you must be prepared for the realities of the medical malpractice system, which may transform your original wishes into legally accepted claims that are more realistic and suitable for a courtroom.[7] For example, you may start out with the goal of making a change in the way a hospital operates ("a system-wide change"), but the limitations of a lawsuit may be a cash settlement and nothing more. Although you have been "compensated," you may be dissatisfied with the result.

Disclosure

One thing that does make patients happier is getting a clear explanation of what happened to them. The public expects physicians to be honest, open, and forthcoming about medical errors. In fact, research shows that people are largely unanimous in wanting full disclosure when medical care goes wrong, including (in order of diminishing priority):[8]

1. A clear statement that an error has occurred
2. An explanation providing full details about the error
3. A sincere apology
4. Reassurances that the something is being done to make sure the error does not happen again
5. Financial compensation for injury, pain, or suffering
6. Accountability on the part of the responsible physician

As you'll notice, financial compensation is almost last on the list. The other items are similar to the extra-legal objectives you just read about. Apparently, most people feel that apologies and full disclosure are more important than financial compensation. If there are other ways to get that disclosure, perhaps you won't need a lawsuit after all.

Good Communication

Disclosure requires communication, but many physicians avoid any contact with patients whom they may have harmed. Often, a lack of communication or a timely response by the physician can be the deciding point that causes patients to seek a malpractice claim.[9]

Here's what frequently may happen: After discharge from the hospital, patients usually call the doctor's office if they're concerned about increasing pain or the wound looking worse. More often than not, the patient doesn't get to speak with the doctor and is just told it is "normal" and to come in for the regularly scheduled visit. If the patient does develop an infection or other complications, she may become bitter, seek revenge, and file a lawsuit. It all comes down to lack of communication and trust in the physician-patient relationship.

Teaching the "3 Rs"

Because lawsuits are so expensive and time consuming, some professional organizations are trying to promote methods to improve communication. For example, the malpractice insurance company COPIC, which serves about 6,000 Colorado and Nebraska physicians, sponsors the "3 Rs Program— Recognize, Respond, and Resolve." Physician members enroll in the program by signing a commitment to receive communication training and follow the 3 Rs technique.[10]

The purpose of the 3 Rs Program is to teach physicians how to facilitate candid, early communication with patients who have experienced an unanticipated medical outcome. They should:

- *Recognize* that a problem has occurred,
- *Respond* to the patient in a timely manner, and
- *Resolve* the situation by communicating empathetically with the patient and arranging for additional care or services the patient may need because of the medical injury.

The idea is that an apology and an upfront financial offer could save the patient/physician relationship and could mean the difference between settlements costing just thousands of dollars and medical lawsuits costing many millions in attorney fees and jury awards. Nevertheless, the 3 Rs Program does not remove a patient's right to pursue legal action. Patients are not required to sign a waiver in order to receive program benefits. If a patient submits a written demand for compensation or pursues a legal route, he or she becomes ineligible for further program benefits at that point.

"Medical Apology Laws"

Similar to the 3 Rs, an increasing number of states have recently taken the lead in trying to curb malpractice cases by encouraging dialog between physicians and patients. Among the most popular and successful state efforts is the passage of so-called "medical apology laws." The laws protect a medical provider who expresses an "apology" to a patient by stipulating that the provider's statements cannot be introduced as evidence against him or her in a subsequent malpractice lawsuit. In other words, if a physician apologizes to you and you then decide to file a lawsuit, that apology cannot be made known to the jury. As of 2011, some 36 states have enacted some form of apology laws or regulations, including California,[11] Florida,[12] Massachusetts,[13] and Texas,[14] among others.

Consider Mediation

What if your doctor hasn't learned his medical 3 Rs and your state doesn't have a medical apology law? That doesn't mean you'll have to file a lawsuit. Consider mediation instead.

In legal situations, mediation is a dispute resolution process in which an impartial third party, known as a "mediator," facilitates negotiations among the parties, with the assistance of their attorneys, to help them reach a mutually acceptable settlement. The major distinction with mediation is that a mediator does not make a decision about the outcome of the case.[15]

Mediation often works well in cases of medical malpractice or negligence where barriers to settlement are personal or emotional (for example, a child dies from a medical error), or where people want to tailor a solution to meet their specific needs or interests (such as a lecture presented in a person's name or some other ongoing way of remembering the person who died or was harmed). Mediation is also an attractive alternative for hospitals and physicians who want a more private forum for resolving disputes instead of the publicity a lawsuit can create.

Voluntary Mediation

Rush Presbyterian-St. Luke's Medical Center in Chicago implemented a voluntary mediation program in 1995 that successfully brought resolution to medical malpractice cases, while lowering the legal costs.[16] Still in use today, their method is different from traditional mediation in that two co-mediators are utilized, instead of a single mediator. Both mediators are expert medical malpractice attorneys, as well as trained mediators. One attorney assists the plaintiff (the injured person) and the other assists the defense (the hospital and/or the doctor).

About one-third of the malpractice suits at Rush Hospital go into the voluntary mediation program each year; 90 percent are successfully settled. Because of its success, the program has served as a model for other hospitals that look for ways to bring patients, doctors, and hospital management together around a table, instead of the courtroom.

Some hospitals are also seeking to integrate co-mediation into a health system's risk management system, so that mediation becomes a first step, rather than the dispute heading straight for the courtroom. In 2004, Philadelphia's Drexel University College of Medicine was the first institution in southeastern Pennsylvania to adopt a formal medical malpractice mediation program. Drexel's program relies on the co-mediation model, consisting of a team of a plaintiff's attorney and a defense malpractice attorney working together.[17]

Mandatory Mediation

To combat rising healthcare costs and legal liability expenses, some hospitals are requiring mandatory mediation. For example, the University of Florida Health Science Center recently completed a preliminary trial of the Florida Patient Safety and Pre-Suit Mediation Program.[18] Before filing a formal lawsuit, the plaintiff and the defendant are required to participate in confidential, non-binding mediation conducted by a neutral third-party mediator.

Arbitration: Praise and Precautions

What would you do after spending many hours in mediation without achieving a reasonable settlement with your doctor or hospital? You've probably read about similar disputes between large employers and their employees. When mediation breaks down, the workers often go on strike. At that point, local officials may insist that both sides move into arbitration.

You may have heard the term arbitration thrown around in the same sentence as mediation and litigation. They're often confused. Simply put, arbitration and mediation are alternatives to litigation (a lawsuit in court). Both arbitration and mediation use a neutral third party. The main difference is that with arbitration, the "arbitrator" generally acts much like a judge. The evidence is presented and argued by both sides (through their attorneys), and the arbitrator issues a decision.

Arbitration has surfaced in the medical context because some doctors and hospitals are using "arbitration clauses" in forms that patients are asked to sign when they agree to medical treatment. By signing, you've agreed to mandatory binding arbitration. That means you've agreed not to sue in court; instead you must go through arbitration.

You've probably seen and signed an arbitration agreement without even realizing it, for example, in your cell phone, rental car, and credit card contracts. Often consumers are unaware that by signing the contract, they have "agreed" to waive their right to a trial. If it's a dispute with your cell phone company, this may seem trivial. However, when the dispute is between you and your doctor or hospital about treatments that affect your health and well-being, you may be signing away more than you think.

Several years ago, the American Arbitration Association, the world's largest arbitration organization, stated publicly that they will no longer hear and decide arbitration agreements dealing with healthcare issues unless the agreement was signed by the patient *after* the dispute arose. In other words, if you signed an agreement mandating arbitration *before* you sustained a medical injury, you should not have to participate in arbitration when you file a lawsuit.

Avoid any possible problem by taking the time to read the fine print before you sign any hospital forms. Be sure that you're not signing away your rights to pursue a legal claim through mediation, lawsuits, or any other form of conflict resolution.

Another Approach: Disclosure-and-Offer

Voluntary mediation and arbitration have shown some success, but have failed to become widely used. Now, some hospitals are trying a new technique called "disclosure-and-offer." This approach links financial compensation to improvements in patient safety.[19]

How this works is that hospitals adopt a practice of being candid (open and sincere) about medical injuries, voluntarily informing patients when an error has occurred and voluntarily compensating anyone who is injured. This disclosure-and-offer approach has been implemented by a handful of hospital systems and liability insurers, building on an early experiment at the Veterans Affairs Hospital in Lexington, Kentucky.[20]

The idea behind disclosing errors to patients and then offering some form of compensation is rooted in a philosophy of hospital risk management. In other words, hospitals hope that being candid about medical injuries, apologizing when appropriate, and providing quick financial compensation will eliminate patients' and families' impulse to sue and will spur institutional learning and safety improvements.[21]

FILE A COMPLAINT

All of the options you've read about so far—lawsuits, mediation, arbitration, and disclosure-and-offer—are used mostly for major medical injuries. But what if you're angry and disgusted about poor care you received in a hospital, even though you have no injuries to show for it? Unfortunately for you, having frustrated expectations does not necessarily imply negligence or a meritorious claim. You can't sue just because you had to wait too long for a bed pan or if you were almost given the wrong medication but the nurse caught the error in time. A mistake with consequences needs to have been made.

Hospitals and doctors are required to follow many healthcare guidelines and standards. If your care falls below that level of quality, the hospital can be penalized by loss of its license or accreditation.

That's where the Joint Commission comes in. Accreditation from the Joint Commission is the premier certification that the best hospitals want to obtain. The Joint Commission's mission is "[t]o continuously improve the safety and quality of care provided to the public through the provision of healthcare accreditation and related services that support performance improvement in healthcare organizations."[22] The Joint Commission's seal of approval is the gold standard in quality of care and best practices. Through the Joint Commission and its certificate programs, patient safety has been pushed forward onto the agendas of hospital boards nationwide.

How to Complain

If your hospital is accredited by the Joint Commission, the administrators have signed an agreement that they will follow medical guidelines and will take action whenever patients register a complaint. So, if you have a complaint about the quality of care at an accredited hospital, go to the Joint Commission website (http://www.jointcommission.org/accreditation/hospitals.aspx) and fill out their simple complaint form.[23] Enter the complaint online or send it by mail, fax, or e-mail.

You may submit your complaint anonymously, but if you provide your name and contact information, the Joint Commission will inform you about any actions taken in response to your complaint, or contact you if additional information is needed. The form also provides a space to write a narrative of the incident and to include a brief overview of your complaint. Just telling your story to "the authorities" may help you feel much better.

Another Approach

Many people do get a satisfactory response from the complaints they file. However, some consumer groups think that mere complaints don't do enough to protect patients' safety. It may require something stronger to motivate hospitals to take patient safety more seriously.[24] That's because, by law, the right to safety cannot be enforced against a physician, but can be used only against a hospital, as an institution which has a duty to ensure patient safety. A case heard by the Pennsylvania Supreme Court expressed this argument more clearly, stating that "Corporate negligence is a doctrine under which the hospital is liable if it fails to uphold the proper standard of care owed to the patient, which is to ensure the patient's safety and well-being while at the hospital."[25]

But how does a patient assert his or her right against a large entity such as a hospital? One idea that's been proposed is to establish hospital care and safety standards. That way, if a hospital fails to meet those standards, it would be liable for damages when complaints are made against individual doctors who jeopardize patients' safety.

One organization that has acted on this is "The 100,000 Lives Campaign" of the Institute for Healthcare Improvement (IHI), which set a goal to have hospitals agree to implement six safety interventions aimed at improving healthcare quality. These procedures include use of rapid response teams, providing reliable care for acute myocardial infarction (heart attack), and preventing central line infections. As the name indicates, the goal is "saving 100,000 lives."[26]

The 100,000 Lives Campaign has become a "standard of care" for hospitals. Those hospitals that haven't participated are left to " . . . explain why particular interventions will not improve patient safety in their institutions."[27] This standard puts the focus on patient safety systems in hospitals, rather than on the actions of individual physicians. That way, hospital boards have a strong incentive to make their environments safer.

PUBLIC DISCLOSURE AND PATIENT EMPOWERMENT

Thanks to the culture of safety generated by consumer groups, the National Practitioner Data Bank (NPDB) was created in 1986, as part of the U.S. Healthcare Quality Improvement Act. The NPDB collects and stores extensive reports about individual doctors' malpractice lawsuits, settlements, and verdicts, along with "other compulsorily reportable actions, such as licensure revocation or suspension, medical staff discipline, and the exclusion of a practitioner from Medicare or Medicaid reimbursement."[28] The good news is that the threat of being reported to the NPDB may improve physicians' behavior. The bad news is that disclosure of NPDB data is strictly limited, so the general public is not permitted to access this important information.

However, some methods are available for consumers to obtain limited information about physician errors. One such mechanism is through investigations performed by Medicare's peer review organization. Thanks to successful federal court cases, Medicare beneficiaries are now able to request investigations by "peer review organizations" as a way to identify substandard physician care. The government is compelled to disclose the results of those investigations.[29]

WHAT I'VE LEARNED AS AN EXPERT WITNESS

Reading my daughter's comprehensive explanation of medical disputes reminds me of cases in which I served as the expert witness for both the defense and the plaintiff.

I can recall cases in which it was very clear to me in reading the patients' discovery that lack of communication by the doctor or other healthcare providers is the single factor that motivates patients to decide to call in the law. You remember from the introduction section of this book how distraught Teri was when she believed she was responsible for her mother's death and how she told us there was little communication with the doctor and so many unanswered questions. Remember, too, she did not call in the law; she just wanted closure and answers.

There are some cases I review that are so obvious—the infection was preventable and for those patients there should be compensation.

I believe as we go forward, good communication through patient empowerment and public disclosure will make our healthcare system safer and more responsive to patients that do become harmed.

You have the empowerment tools in this book and you have the facts about the law and your options. Use both wisely.

My Closing Thoughts:
Partnership and Forgiveness

It is my hope that by reading this book, you have become empowered to take the steps you need, so you won't wind up with a healthcare-associated infection, and you won't have to consider a lawsuit. However, we must face the fact that despite all efforts, infections sometimes do occur. How you handle that situation will affect not only you and your family but also could have an impact on our entire healthcare system.

If you think that sounds too dramatic, take a moment to reflect on the story of Kerry O'Connell. A botched surgery on his injured arm, which lead to a 2 year struggle with methicillin-resistant *Staphylococcus aureus* (MRSA). Yes, he was angry and aggrieved, but he used his difficult experience to make positive changes in the medical system by helping to pass laws that benefit many people. There is no better way to end this chapter about the law than to share Kerry's own words, describing his battle to understand "Why me?" and then to move on and help others:

> *I believe that understanding <u>why</u> is the crucial first step towards ultimate forgiveness. All of us are highly imperfect beings who make mistakes every day. The truth is never hard to understand. Doctors' greatest weakness is that they don't understand that true forgiveness transforms both parties. It is a growth experience far more valuable than maintaining any mythic reputation [that doctors are perfect].*

> *What can be done to dispel the myth? Our most valuable tool may be to be absolutely honest with doctors and strongly encourage them to be honest with us. When you encounter honesty, cherish it, praise it, and tell the world about it, for true honesty is quite rare. The two*

things that all doctors should learn early in their profession are that no amount of cash can replace competent compassionate care and that honesty can heal the soul when nothing can heal the body!

[At my] much anticipated and dreaded meeting with my original doctor, as much as I pressed, he didn't want to talk about the details of what went wrong. So I explained what I thought happened. He hung his head and nodded [in agreement]. He did admit that a lot of people messed up . . . badly. He explained that it was the second worst thing that has ever happened to him in his career and that he lost a lot of sleep over me.

His practice doesn't do any more plunge incisions and will never use another elbow fixator [the surgery that permanently damaged Kerry's arm]. *The doctor excitedly explained a new system of injecting Botox into the elbow to prevent the buildup of scar tissue. I sat there and realized he has no interest at all in educating the orthopedic world about my problem, and what could go wrong, which drives me absolutely insane.*

I told him my theory that God caused this to teach me a few things about life. He said God taught him a lot also. Though I still didn't know why this tragedy happened, I told him that I forgave him, he hugged me, the attorneys were touched (really). 1 can only hope that he feels better . . . .

Glossary

Acute illness—A sudden and severe condition.

Acute care hospital—A hospital facility that has the staff and equipment to provide short-term treatment of acute conditions (*see* Acute illness).

Ambulatory surgery centers—Medical facilities that specialize in elective same-day or outpatient surgical procedures. (Also known as outpatient surgery centers)

Antibiotic—A medication that kills or inhibits the growth of susceptible microorganisms.

Antiseptic agent—A substance such as alcohol or chlorhexidine, that inactivates microorganisms (antimicrobial action) or inhibits their growth on living tissues.

Arbitration—A dispute resolution process in which an impartial third party (the arbitrator) listens to evidence presented by attorneys for each side and then issues a decision.

Assisted living facility—A residential housing setting that provides limited personal care assistance, meal services, and activity programs.

Bacteria—A type of single-cell microorganism, some of which cause disease.

Catheter—A flexible tube available in many sizes that is used to inject fluids or medicines and to remove blood and other body fluids.

Central venous catheter—A flexible tube inserted through the skin of the neck, chest, or groin into a large vein that carries blood directly toward the heart. (Sometimes called a "central line")

Chronic illness—A lasting or prolonged condition.

Colonization—Growth and multiplication of bacteria or viruses, but without patients having yet developed any symptoms of illness.

Contamination—Presence of bacteria and other microorganisms on the hands, other body surfaces, and objects.

Culture—In medical care, taking a sample of tissue or fluid from a patient, placing it in a flat covered dish containing a nutrient mixture, and checking for growth of bacteria or viruses.

Damages—Legal compensation for harm or injury.

Defendant—The person accused of wrongdoing in a legal complaint.

Defense attorney—A lawyer representing a defendant.

Epidemic—A significant increase in the number of cases of a disease, above the usual level of occurrence in that medical facility or community.

Foley catheter—A tube that is inserted into the urinary bladder in order to drain urine out into a plastic collection bag.

Gloves (medical)—Disposable hand coverings used during medical and surgical procedures may be non-sterile or sterile with sterile packaging.

Hand hygiene—Any action taken to cleanse the hands.

Hand sanitizer—A liquid, gel, or foam, usually containing alcohol, that is designed for application to the hands to inactivate microorganisms and/or temporarily reduce their growth.

Handwashing—Cleansing hands with water and plain or antimicrobial soap, to remove dirt, organic material, and/or microorganisms.

Healthcare-associated infections—Infectious illnesses that patients develop during or after their stay in a hospital or healthcare facility and that were not present at the time they were admitted, but were caused by in-hospital transmission of bacteria, viruses, or other microorganisms. (Also called hospital-associated infections or nosocomial infections)

Healthcare directive—A written legal document that allows a person to appoint another person (agent) to make healthcare decisions should he or she be unable to make or communicate decisions.

Healthcare worker—Any paid or unpaid person working in a healthcare setting, including (but not limited to) physicians, nurses, nursing assistants, therapists, and technicians.

High-low agreement—A legal guarantee that the plaintiff in a medical lawsuit will receive at least some minimum amount of money (the "low"), but not more than a capped amount (the "high").

Hygiene—Cleanliness that promotes health and well-being.

Informed consent—Process of giving written permission to undergo a test or procedure, indicating that the signer understands why the procedure is needed, and the risks and benefits of the potential result.

Inpatient—A person who has been formally admitted to a hospital or other health facility and is discharged after one or more days.

Intensive care unit (ICU)—A specialized hospital unit where patients receive close monitoring and continuous care.

Intravenous catheter—A thin, flexible tube inserted through the skin into a vein, used to deliver fluids and medications directly into the bloodstream.

Invasive—In surgical procedures, entering the body through an incision in the skin (surgical cut) or by insertion of medical instruments.

IV or intravenous infusion—Administration of liquid medications, blood, or nutritional solutions directly into the bloodstream through a catheter tube that is inserted into a vein.

Lawsuit—A complaint against an individual or individuals that is entered into court proceedings for settlement.

Long-term care facility—An institution that provides healthcare to people who are chronically disabled and require continued assistance with daily activities.

Malpractice (medical)—Improper or negligent treatment by a medical professional or facility that does not meet accepted standards of practice and results in harm to a patient.

Mediation—A dispute resolution process in which an impartial third party (the mediator) facilitates negotiations among the parties, with their attorneys, to help them reach a settlement.

Meningitis—Bacterial infection of membranes covering the brain and spinal cord.

Microorganism—A bacterium, virus, or other living thing that is too small to be seen by the naked eye.

Negligence—Conduct that does not meet the standards of behavior established by law for the protection of others against unreasonable risk of harm.

Nosocomial infections—*See* Healthcare-associated infections.

Nursing home—A type of long-term care facility with an organized professional staff that provides continuous nursing care and other services to inpatients who have chronic illnesses.

Outpatient—A person who receives care at a hospital or other health facility without being admitted to stay overnight or longer.

Peripheral venous catheter—Flexible tube that is inserted through the skin and into a vein in the arm or leg, for use in administering fluids and medication directly into the bloodstream. (Also called a "peripheral line")

Plaintiff—The person ("complainant") making a claim of injury and bringing the complaint into a court of law.

Prosecutor—The lawyer (a district attorney, state's attorney, or U.S. attorney) who investigates and tries criminal cases.

Sepsis—Severe bacterial infection in the bloodstream and body tissues that causes life-threatening symptoms. (Also referred to as septicemia or "blood poisoning")

Surgical site infection—An infection of the surgical wound, or any organ or any area of the body that was contacted during surgery.

Urinary catheter—A long, thin, flexible tube inserted through the urethra used to drain urine out of the bladder and down into a plastic collection bag.

Ventilator—A machine (also called a respirator) that pushes air into the lungs through a breathing tube placed in the trachea (the "windpipe"), used to provide oxygen for people who can't breathe well enough on their own.

Visibly soiled hands—Hands showing dirt or body fluids that are readily observable.

References

INTRODUCTION

1. Klevens, R. M., J. R. Edwards, C. L. Richards, T. C. Hortan, R. P. Gaynes, D. A. Pollock, D. M. Cardo. 2007. Estimating healthcare associated infections and deaths in U.S. hospitals. *Public Health Rep* 122:160-6. http://www.cdc.gov/ncidod/dhqp/pdf/nicpad/infections_deaths.pdf (accessed July 5, 2011).
2. Scott, R. D II. March 2009. The Direct Medical Costs of Healthcare-Associated Infections in U.S. Hospitals and the Benefits of Prevention. Division of Healthcare Quality Promotion, National Center for Preparedness, Detection, and Control of Infectious Diseases, Coordinating Center for Infectious Diseases, Centers for Disease Control and Prevention. http://www.cdc.gov/ncidod/dhqp/pdf/Scott_CostPaper.pdf (accessed May 15, 2010).
3. McGuckin, M. 2004. *What to Do Before—A Consumer's Guide to Handwashing*. Ardmore, PA: MMI.
4. Quaraishi, Z., and M. B. McGuckin. 1984. Duration of hand-washing frequency in two intensive care units. *Am J Infect Control* 12:83-7.
5. McGuckin, M. B., and E. Abrutyn. 1979. A surveillance method for early detection of nosocomial outbreaks. *Am J Infect Control* 7:18-21.
6. Kaplan, L. M., and M. B. McGuckin. 1986. Increasing handwashing compliance with more accessible sinks. *Am J Infect Control* 14:408-10.
7. McGuckin, M., R. Waterman, and J. Govednik. 2009. Hand hygiene compliance in the United States. A one-year multicenter collaboration

using product/volume usage measurement and feedback. *Am J Med Qual* 24:205-13.

8. McGuckin, M., R. Waterman, L. Porten, et al. 1999. Patient education model for increasing handwashing compliance. *Am J Infect Control* 27:309-14.

9. McGuckin, M., R. Waterman, J. Storr, et al. 2001. Evaluation of patient empowering hand hygiene programme in UK. *J Hosp Infect* 48:222-7.

10. McGuckin, M., A. Shubin, P. McBride, et al. 2006. The effect of random voice hand hygiene messages delivered by medical, nursing, and infection control staff on hand hygiene compliance in intensive care. *Am J Infect Control* 34:673-5.

CHAPTER 1

1. U.S. Department of Health and Human Services, National Institutes of Health, National Institute of Allergy and Infectious Diseases. 2006. Understanding Microbes in Sickness and in Health. NIH Publication No. 06-4914. http://www.niaid.nih.gov/topics/microbes/Documents/microbesbook.pdf (accessed May 15, 2010).

2. National Institutes of Health, National Institute of Allergy and Infectious Diseases. 1999. Emerging and Re-Emerging Infectious Diseases. NIH Curriculum Supplement Series—Grades 9-12. Colorado Springs, CO: BSCS and Videodiscovery, Inc. http://science.education.nih.gov/supplements/nih1/diseases/default.htm (accessed May 18, 2010).

3. Snow, V., C. Mottur-Pilson, and R. Gonzales. 2001. Principles of appropriate antibiotic use for treatment of nonspecific upper respiratory tract infections in adults. *Ann Inter Med* 134:487-9.

4. Centers for Disease Control and Prevention. 2002. Guideline for hand hygiene in health-care settings: Recommendations of the healthcare infection control practices advisory committee and the HICPAC/SHEA/APIC/IDSA hand hygiene task force. *Morb Mortal Wkly Rep* 51(No. RR-16):1-30.

5. U.S. Department of Health and Human Services, National Institutes of Health, National Institute of Allergy and Infectious Diseases. 2007. Understanding the Immune System: How It Works. NIH Publication No. 07-5423. http://www.niaid.gov/topics/ImmuneSystem/Documents/theimmunesystem.pdsf (accessed May 15, 2010).

6. Todar, K. 2008. Colonization and invasion by bacterial pathogens. In *Todar's Online Textbook of Bacteriology*. http://www.textbookofbacteriology.net (accessed May 17, 2010).

7. Trüper, H. G. 1999. How to name a prokaryote? Etymological considerations, proposals and practical advice in prokaryote nomenclature. *FEMS Microbiol Rev* 23:231–49.
8. Centers for Disease Control and Prevention. Emerging Infectious Diseases: Scientific Nomenclature. http://www.cdc.gov/ncidod/eid/StyleGuide/scientific_nomenclature.htm (accessed November 4, 2011).
9. Madoff, L. C., and D. L. Kasper. 2008. Infectious Diseases, Section 1, Chapter113. Introduction to infectious diseases: Host-pathogen interactions. In *Harrison's Principles of Internal Medicine*, 17th ed. New York: McGraw-Hill Professional.
10. World Health Organization. 2009. *WHO Guidelines on Hand Hygiene in Healthcare*. Geneva: WHO Press.

CHAPTER 2

1. Horan, T. C., M. Andrus, and M. A. Dudeck. 2008. CDC/NHSN surveillance definition of healthcare-associated infection and criteria for specific types of infections in the acute care setting. *Am J Infect Control* 36:309–32.
2. U.S. Department of Health & Human Services. 2009. HHS Action Plan to Prevent Healthcare-Associated Infections. U.S. Department of Health & Human Services, Washington, DC. http://www.hhs.gov/ophs/initiatives/hai/infection.html (accessed June 3, 2010).
3. Klevens, R. M., J. R. Edwards, C. L. Richards, T. C. Hortan, R. Gaynes, D. Pollock, D. Cardo. 2007. Estimating healthcare associated infections and deaths in U.S. hospitals. *Public Health Rep* 122:160–6. www.cdc.gov/ncidod/dhqp/pdf/nicpad/infections_deaths.pdf (accessed May 7, 2011).
4. Yokoe, D. S., L. A. Mermel, D. J. Anderson, K. M. Arias, H. Burstin, D. P. Calfee, S. E. Coffin, E. R. Dubberke, V. Fraser, D. N. Gerding, et al. 2008. A compendium of strategies to prevent healthcare-associated infections in acute care hospitals. *Infect Control Hosp Epidemiol* 29:S12–S21.
5. National Healthcare Quality Report, 2009. U.S. 2010. Department of Health and Human Services, Agency for Healthcare Research and Quality, Publication #10-0003. http://www.ahrq.gov/qual/qrdr09.htm (accessed May 28, 2010).
6. Scott, R. D. II. 2009. The direct medical costs of healthcare-associated infections in U.S. hospitals and the benefits of prevention. Centers for Disease Control and Prevention. http://www.cdc.gov/ncidod/dhqp/pdf/Scott_Cost.Paper.pdf (accessed October 29, 2010).

7. Mobile phone is a hygiene risk, study says. 2010. Infection Control Today. http://infectioncontroltoday.com/news/2010/08/mobile-phone-is-a-hygiene-risk-study-says.aspx (accessed May 9, 2011).
8. Yokoe, D. S., and D. Classen. 2008. Improving patient safety through infection control: A new healthcare imperative. *Infect Control Hosp Epidemiol* 29:S3–S11.
9. Facts about Joint Commission accreditation and certification. 2011. The Joint Commission, Oakbrook Terrace, IL. http://www.jointcommission.org/facts_about_joint_commission_accreditation_and_certification (accessed May 9, 2011).
10. State legislation and initiatives on healthcare-associated infections. 2010. Committee to Reduce Infection Deaths. http://hospitalinfection.org/legislation.shtml (accessed May 9, 2011).
11. Health facility acquired infections reporting initiative reports: 2011 Annual Report. Colorado Department of Public Health and Environment. http://www.cdphe.state.co.us/hf/PatientSafety/HFAI/reports.html (accessed May 9, 2011).
12. McGuckin, M., R. Waterman, and A. Shubin. 2006. Consumer attitudes about healthcare-associated infections and hand hygiene. *Am J Med Qual* 21:342-6.
13. Cardo, D., T. Horan, M. Andrus, M. Dembinski, J. Edwards, G. Peavy, J. Tolston, and D. Wagner. 2004. National Nosocomial Infections Surveillance (NNIS) System Report, data summary from January 1992 through June 2004, issued October 2004. *Am J Infect Control* 32:470–85.

CHAPTER 3

1. Centers for Disease Control and Prevention. 2010. Definition of MRSA. Centers for Disease Control and Prevention. http://www.cdc.gov/mrsa/definition/index.html (accessed August 9, 2010).
2. National Institute of Allergy and Infectious Diseases. 2011. Antimicrobial (Drug) Resistance: Methicillin-resistant *Staphylococcus aureus* (MRSA). National Institute of Allergy and Infectious Diseases. http://www.niaid.nih.gov/topics/antimicrobialresistance/examples/mrsa/Pages/default.aspx (accessed January 5, 2012).
3. Carriere, M. D., and C. F. Decker. 2008. MRSA: An evolving pathogen. *Dis Mon* 54:751-5.
4. Chavez, T. T., and C. F. Decker. 2008. Healthcare-associated MRSA versus community-associated MRSA. *Dis Mon* 54:763-8.
5. Johnson, M. D., and C. F. Decker. 2008. Antimicrobial agents in treatment of MRSA infections. *Dis Mon* 54:793-800.

6. Centers for Disease Control and Prevention. 2011. FAQs About MRSA. Centers for Disease Control and Prevention, SHEA/IDSA HAI Prevention Compendium. http://cdc.gov/ncidod/dhqp/NAI_shea_idsa.html (accessed May 10, 2011).

7. Herigon, J. C., A. L. Hersh, J. S. Gerber, T. E. Zaoutis, and J. G. Newland. 2010. Antibiotic management of *Staphylococcus aureus* infections in U.S. children's hospitals, 1999–2008. *Pediatrics* 125:e1294–e1300. http://pediatrics.aappublications.org.cgi/search?sortspec=relevance&fulltext=Herigon (accessed May 17, 2010).

8. Zeller, J. L., A. E. Burke, and R. M. Glass. 2007. MRSA Infections. *J Am Med Assoc* 298:1826. http://jama.ama-assn.org/cgi/reprint/298/15/1826.pdf (accessed July 23, 2010).

9. Murray, B. E. 1998. Diversity among multidrug-resistant enterococci. *Emerg Infect Dis* 4:37–48. Updated February 23, 2010, http://www.cdc.gov/ncidod/eid/vol4no1/murray.htm (accessed July 21, 2010).

10. National Institute of Allergy and Infectious Diseases. 2008. Antimicrobial (Drug) Resistance: Vancomycin-resistant *enterococci* (VRE). National Institute of Allergy and Infectious Diseases. http://www.niaid.nih.gov/topics/antimicrobialresistance/examples/vre/Pages/default.aspx (accessed July 23, 2010).

11. Dubberke, E. R., D. N. Gerding, D. Classen, et al. 2008. Strategies to prevent *Clostridium difficile* infections in acute care hospitals. *Infect Control Hosp Epidemiol* 29:S81–S92.

12. Torpy, J. M., C. Lynm, and R. M. Glass. 2009. *Clostridium difficile* colitis. *J Am Med Assoc* 301:988.

13. Centers for Disease Control and Prevention/Infectious Disease Society of America. 2010. FAQs About *Clostridium Difficile*. Centers for Disease Control and Prevention/Infectious Disease Society of America, HAI Prevention Compendium. http://cdc.gov/ncidod/dhqp/HAI_shea_idsa.html (accessed July 7, 2010).

14. Mayfield, J. L. 2010. Preventing *Clostridium difficile* infection (CDI)—An infection preventionist's perspective. Centers for Disease Control and Prevention Safe Healthcare blog. http://blogs.cdc.gov/safehealthcare/?page_id=358 (accessed July 14, 2010).

15. McDonald, L. C. 2010. Dr. Cliff on tackling *C. difficile*—Part 1 of 3. Centers for Disease Control and Prevention Safe Healthcare blog. http://blogs.cdc.gov/safehealthcare/?page_id=358 (accessed June 4, 2010).

16. McFarland, L. V. 2009. Renewed interest in a difficult disease: *Clostridium difficile* infections—Epidemiology and current treatment strategies. *Curr Opin Gastroenterol* 25:24–35.

17. Overview of healthcare-associated MRSA. 2003. Centers for Disease Control and Prevention. http://www.cdc.gov/ncidod/dhqp/ar_mrsa.html (accessed July 21, 2010).
18. Kelly, C. P., and J. T. LaMont. 2008. *Clostridium difficile*—More difficult than ever. *N Engl J Med* 359:1932–40.
19. Yong, D., M. A. Toleman, C. G. Giske, H. S. Cho, K. Sundman, K. Lee, and T. R. Walsh. 2009. Characterization of a new metallo-ß-lactamase gene, *bla* (NDM-1), and a novel erythromycin esterase gene carried on a unique genetic structure in *Klebsiella pneumoniae* sequence type 14 from India. *Antimicrob Agents Chemother* 53:5046–54.
20. Wertheim, H. F., M. C. Vos, H. A. Boelens, A. Voss, C. M. Vandenbroucke-Grauls, M. H. Meester, J. A. Kluytmans, P. H. van Keulen, and H. A. Verbrugh. 2004. Low prevalence of methicillin-resistant *Staphylococcus aureus* (MRSA) at hospital admission in the Netherlands: The value of search and destroy and restrictive antibiotic use. *J Hosp Infect* 56:321–5.
21. Fishman, N. 2010. Dr. Fishman's Top 5: Appropriate antibiotic use. Centers for Disease Control and Prevention Safe Healthcare blog. http://blogs.cdc.gov/safehealthcare/?page =405 (accessed July 14, 2010).
22. McGuckin, M., R. Waterman, and J. Govednik. 2009. Hand hygiene compliance rates in the United States—A one-year multicenter collaboration using product/volume usage measurement and feedback. *Am J Med Qual* 24:205–13.

CHAPTER 4

1. Guinan, M. E., M. McGuckin-Guinan, and A. Sevareid. 1997. Who washes hands after using the bathroom? *Am J Infect Control* 25:424–5.
2. Bayer Pharmaceutical Division and Wirthlin Worldwide Research. 1996. Handwashing survey. Fact sheet distributed at American Society for Microbiology Annual Meeting, New Orleans.
3. Heseltine, P. 2001. Why don't doctors and nurses wash their hands? *Infect Control Hosp Epidemiol* 22:199–200.
4. Quraishi, Z. A., M. McGuckin, and F. X. Blais. 1984. Duration of hand-washing in intensive care units: A descriptive study. *Am J Infect Control* 12:83–7.
5. WHO. 2009. *WHO Guidelines on Hand Hygiene in Healthcare*. Geneva, Switzerland: WHO Press.
6. Pisipati, S., D. Bassett, and I. Pearce. 2009. Do neckties and pens act as vectors of hospital-associated infections? *BJU Int* 103:1604–5.
7. Merlin, M. A., M. L. Wong, P. W. Pryor, K. Rynn, A. Marques-Baptista, R. Perritt, C. Stanescu, and T. Fallon. 2009. Prevalence of methicillin-resistant

Staphylococcus aureus on the stethoscopes of emergency medical service providers. *Prehosp Emerg Care* 13:71–4.

8. Mehta, A. K., J. S. Halvosa, C. V. Gould, and J. P. Steinberg. 2010. Efficacy of alcohol-based hand rubs in the disinfection of stethoscopes. *Infect Control Hosp Epidemiol* 31:870–2.

9. The Joint Commission Center for Transforming Healthcare. Facts about the hand hygiene project. http://www.centerfortransforminghealthcare. org/projects/about_hand_hygiene_project.aspx (accessed May 13, 2011).

10. World Health Organization. Hand Hygiene: Why, How & When? brochure, revised August 2009.

11. Berg, S. Z. Good reasons for hand-wringing over handwashing. *Insight* Magazine, March 2, 2004.

12. Centers for Disease Control and Prevention. Precautions to prevent the spread of MRSA in healthcare settings. http://www.cdc.gov/mrsa/ prevent/healthcare/precautions.html (accessed May 13, 2011).

13. McGuckin, M., and A. Torress-Cook. 2009. Interventional patient hygiene for the wound care professional. *Adv Skin Wound Care* 22:416–20.

14. Boyce, J. 2009. New approaches to decontamination of rooms after patients are discharged. *Infect Control Hosp Epidemiol* 30:515–7.

CHAPTER 5

1. World Health Organization. 2009. *WHO Guidelines on Hand Hygiene in Healthcare*. Geneva, Switzerland: World Health Organization.

2. Lau, D. H. 2002. Patient empowerment: A patient-centered approach to improve care. *Hong Kong Med J* 8:372–4.

3. McGuckin, M., J. Storr, Y. Longtin, B. Allegranzi, and D. Pittet. 1997. Patient empowerment and multimodal hand hygiene promotion: A win-win strategy. *Am J Med Qual* 25:424–5.

4. Kohn, L., J. M. Corrigan, and M. S. Donaldson, eds. 2000. *To Err Is Human: Building a Safer Health System*. Washington, DC: National Academies Press.

5. McGlynn, E. A., S. M. Asch, J. Adams, et al. 2003. The quality of healthcare delivered to adults in the United States. *N Engl J Med* 348:2635–45.

6. Landrigan, C. P., G. J. Parry, C. B. Bones, et al. 2010. Temporal trends in rates of patient harm resulting from medical care. *N Engl J Med* 363:2124–34.

7. Longtin, Y., H. Sax, L. L. Leape, et al. 2010. Patient participation: Current knowledge and applicability to patient safety. *Mayo Clin Proc* 85:53–62.

8. Stewart, M. 1995. Effective physician-patient communication and health outcomes: A review. *Can Med Assoc J* 152:1423–33.

9. Guinan, J., M. McGuckin, A. Shubin, and J. Tighe. 2005. A descriptive review of malpractice claims for healthcare-associated infections in Philadelphia. *Am J Infect Control* 33:310–2.

10. Bredart, A., C. Boulleuc, and S. Dolbeault. 2005. Doctor-patient communication and satisfaction with care in oncology. *Curr Opin Oncol* 17:351–4.

11. McGuckin, M., R. Waterman, and A. Shubin. 2006. Consumer attitudes about healthcare-associated infections and hand hygiene. *Am J Med Qual* 21:342–6.

12. Clancy, C. M. Why it's wise to use a health advocate. Agency for Healthcare Research and Quality, U.S. Department of Health & Human Services, July 6, 2010. http://www.ahrq.gov/consumer/cc/cc070610.htm (accessed July 6, 2010).

13. Shaw, D. A direct advance on advance directives. *Bioethics*. Epub ahead of print at http://www.ncbi.nlm.nih.gov/pubmed/21133977 (accessed December 9, 2010).

14. Sabatino, C. P. 2010. The evolution of healthcare advance planning law and policy. *Milbank Q* 88:211–39.

15. Schwartz, L. 2002. Is there an advocate in the house? The role of healthcare professionals in patient advocacy. *J Med Ethics* 28:37–40.

16. Clancy, C. Consumer/Quality Insider: Family health advocacy. Healthcare 411 (audio transcript) http://www.healthcare411.ahrq.gov/transcript.aspx?id=101 (accessed December 13, 2010).

17. Nelson, J. What is a hospitalist? Society of Hospital Medicine blog, posted February 2, 2010. http://blogs.hospitalmedicine.org/SHMPracti ceManagementBlog/?p=206 (accessed December 9, 2010).

18. Wachter, R. M., and L. Goldman. 2002. The hospitalist movement 5 years later. *J Am Med Assoc* 287:487–94.

19. Vasilevskis, E. E., R. Knebel, A. Dudley, et al. 2010. Cross-sectional analysis of hospitalist prevalence and quality of care in California. *J Hosp Med* 5:200–7.

20. Krist, A. H., and S. H. Woolf. 2011. A vision for patient-centered health information systems. *J Am Med Assoc* 305:300–1.

21. Paasche-Orlow, M. K., D. M. Jacob, M. Hochhauser, et al. 2009. National survey of patients' bill of rights statutes. *J Gen Intern Med* 24:489–4.

22. American Medical Association. Patient Physician Relationship Topics: Informed Consent.http://www.ama-assn.org/ama/pub/physician-resources/

legal-topics/patient-physician-relationship-topics/informed-consent.shtml
(accessed December 9, 2010).

CHAPTER 6

1. McGuckin, M., A. Shubin, and M. Hujcs. 2008 Interventional patient hygiene model: Infection control and nursing share responsibility for patient safety. *Am J Infect Control* 36:59–62.
2. Nabili, S. T. Inability to urinate. WebMD, emedicinehealth, 3/3/2010. http://www.emedicinehealth.com/inability_to_urinate/article_em.htm (accessed June 2, 2010).
3. Centers for Disease Control and Prevention. 2009. An overview of catheter-associated urinary tract infections (UTI). Centers for Disease Control and Prevention, Division of Healthcare Quality and Promotion. http://www.cdc.gov/ncidod/dhqp/dpac_uti.html (accessed June 3, 2010).
4. Urinary catheters. MedlinePlus Medical Encyclopedia. http://www.nlm.nih.gov/medlineplus/ency/article/003981.htm (accessed June 19, 2010).
5. Society of Critical Care Medicine. Urinary drainage. http://www.icu-usa.com/tour/procedures/foley.htm (accessed June 23, 2010).
6. Gould, C. V., C. A. Umscheid, R. K. Agarwal, G. Kuntz, and D. A. Pegues; the Healthcare Infection Control Practices Advisory Committee. 2009. Guideline for Prevention of Catheter-Associated Urinary Tract Infections 2009. Division of Healthcare Quality Promotion, Centers for Disease Control and Prevention. http://www.cdc.gov/ncidod/dhqp/dpac_uri_pc.html (accessed June 3, 2010).
7. Lo, E., L. Nicolle, D. Classen, et al. 2008. SHEA/IDSA Practice Recommendation: Strategies to prevent catheter-associated urinary tract infections in acute care hospitals. *Infect Control Hosp Epidemiol* 29:S41–S50.
8. Chihara, S., K. J. Popovich, R. A. Weinstein, et al. 2010. *Staphylococcus aureus* bacteriuria as a prognosticator for outcome of *Staphylococcus aureus* bacteremia: A case-control study. *BMC Infect Dis* 10:225.
9. Saint, S., J. A. Meddings, D. Calfee, et al. 2009. Catheter-associated urinary tract infection and the Medicare rule changes. *Ann Intern Med* 150:877–84.
10. World Health Organization. 2009. *WHO Guidelines on Hand Hygiene in Healthcare.* Geneva: World Health Organization Press.
11. Saint, S., C. P. Kowalski, S. R. Kaufman, et al. 2008. Preventing hospital-associated urinary tract infection in the United States: A national study. *Clin Infect Dis* 46:243–50.

12. Centers for Disease Control and Prevention's FAQs (Frequently Asked Questions) About Catheter-Associated Urinary Tract Infection (one of 6 patient guides about hospital-associated infections). http://www.cdc.gov/ncidod/dhqp/HAI_shea_idsa.html (accessed June 24, 2010).

13. Meddings, J., M. A. Rogers, M. Macy, et al. 2010. Systematic review and meta-analysis: Reminder systems to reduce catheter-associated urinary tract infections and urinary catheter use in hospitalized patients. *Clin Infect Dis* 51:550–60.

14. Cornia, P. B., and B. A. Lipsky. 2008. Indwelling urinary catheters in hospitalized patients: When in doubt, pull it out. *Infect Control Hosp Epidemiol* 29:820–2.

15. Peleg, A. Y., and D. C. Hooper. 2010. Hospital-associated infections due to gram-negative bacteria. *N Engl J Med* 362:1804–13.

CHAPTER 7

1. National Heart Lung and Blood Institute. What is pneumonia? http://nhlbi.nih.gov/health/dci/Diseases/pnu/pnu_all.html (accessed December 30, 2010).

2. File, T. M. Jr., and T. J. Marrie. 2010. Burden of community-acquired pneumonia in North American Adults. *Postgrad Med* 122:130–41.

3. Ruhnke, G. W., M. Coca-Perraillon, B. T. Kitch, and D. M. Cutler. 2011. Marked reduction in 30-day mortality among elderly patients with community-acquired pneumonia. *Am J Med* 124:171–8.e1.

4. World Health Organization. New and Under-utilized Vaccines Implementation (NUVI): *Streptococcus pneumoniae* (Pneumococcus). http://www.who.int/nuvi/pneumococcus/en/index.html (accessed December 29, 2010).

5. Klevens, R. M., J. R. Edwards, C. L. Richards, T. C. Hortan, R. P. Gaynes, D. A. Pollock, and D. M. Cardo. 2007. Estimating healthcare-associated infections and deaths in U.S. hospitals, 2002. *Public Health Rep* 122:160–6.

6. Eber, M. R., R. Laxminarayan, E. N. Perencevich, and A. Malani. 2010. Clinical and economic outcomes attributable to healthcare-associated sepsis and pneumonia. *Arch Intern Med* 170:347–53.

7. Utter, G. H., J. Cuny, P. Sama, et al. 2010. Detection of postoperative respiratory failure: How predictive is the Agency for Healthcare Research and Quality's Patient Safety Indicator? *J Am Coll Surg* 211:347–54.

8. National Heart Lung and Blood Institute. What is a ventilator? http://www.nhlbi.nih.gov/health/dci/Diseases/vent/vent_all.html (accessed December 30, 2010).

9. Ibrahim, E. H., L. Tracy, C. Hill, et al. 2001. The occurrence of ventilator-associated pneumonia in a community hospital: Risk factors and clinical outcomes. *Chest* 120:555–61.
10. American Thoracic Society. 2005. Guidelines for the management of adults with hospital-associated, ventilator-associated, and healthcare-associated pneumonia. *Am J Crit Care Med* 171:388–416.
11. Rello, J., J. A. Paiva, J. Baraibar, et al. 2001. International conference for the development of consensus on the diagnosis and treatment of ventilator-associated pneumonia. *Chest* 120:955–70.
12. Coffin, S. E., M. Klompas, D. Classen, et al. 2008. Strategies to prevent ventilator-associated pneumonia in acute care hospitals (SHEA/IDSA Practice Recommendation). *Infect Control Hosp Epidemiol* 29(Suppl 1): S31–S40.
13. Berwick, D. M., D. R. Calkins, C. J. McCannon, and A. D. Hackbarth. 2006. The 100,000 Lives Campaign: Setting a goal and a deadline for improving healthcare quality. *J Am Med Assoc* 295:324–7.
14. Baylor Regional Medical Center at Plano (BRMCP). Zero tolerance: The VAP Prevention Initiative. http://www.hpoe.org/PDFs/Case%20Study--Baylor%20Regional.pdf (accessed May 6, 2011).
15. Institute for Healthcare Improvement. Implement the Ventilator Bundle. http://www.ihi.org/IHI/Topics/CriticalCare/IntensiveCare/Changes/ImplementtheVentilatorBundle.htm (accessed November 15, 2010).
16. Cutler, C. J., and N. Davis. 2005. Improving oral care in patients receiving mechanical ventilation. *Am J Crit Care* 14:389–94.
17. van Nieuwenhoven, C. A., C. Vandenbroucke-Grauls, F. H. van Tiel, et al. 2006. Feasibility and effects of the semirecumbent position to prevent ventilator-associated pneumonia: A randomized study. *Crit Care Med* 34:396–402.

CHAPTER 8

1. de Vries, E. N., H. A. Prins, R. Crolla, A. J. den Outer, G. van Andel, S. H. van Helden, W. S. Schlack, et al. 2010. Effect of a comprehensive surgical safety system on patient outcomes. *N Engl J Med* 363:1928–37.
2. de Vries, E. N., M. A. Ramrattan, S. M. Smorenburg, D. J. Gouma, and M. A. Boermeester. 2008. The incidence and nature of in-hospital adverse events: A systematic review. *Qual Safe Healthcare* 17:216–23.
3. Kirkland, K. B., J. P. Briggs, S. L. Trivette, W. E. Wilkinson, D. J. Sexton. 1999. The impact of surgical-site infections in the 1990s: Attributable mortality, excess length of hospitalization, and extra costs. *Infect Control Hosp Epidemiol* 20:725–30.

4. World Health Organization. Safe surgery saves lives: The second global patient safety challenge. http://www.who.int/patientsafety/safesurgery/en/ (accessed February 1, 2011).

5. Weiser, T. G., A. B. Haynes, G. Dziekan, W. R. Berry, S. R. Lipsitz, A. A. Gawande; Safe Surgery Saves Lives Investigators and Study Group. 2010. Effect of a 19-item surgical safety checklist during urgent operations in a global patient population. *Ann Surg* 251:976–80.

6. Humphreys, H. 2009. Preventing surgical site infection. Where now? *J Hosp Infect* 73:316–22.

7. Lai, P. B. S. 2011. Quality of surgery. *Surg Pract* 15:1.

8. Russell, T. R. 2008. *I Need an Operation...Now What?* Chicago, IL: American College of Surgeons and Thomson Healthcare.

9. The Consumer Assessment of Healthcare Providers and Systems Consortium. 2010. CAHPS surgical care survey. Agency for Healthcare Research and Quality. https://www.cahps.ahrq.gov/content/products/sc/PROD_SC_Surgical_Care.asp (accessed February 2, 2011).

10. Torpy, J. M., A. Burke, and R. M. Glass. 2005. Wound infections. *J Am Med Assoc* 294:2212.

11. Wenzel, R. P. 2010. Minimizing surgical-site infections. *N Engl J Med* 362:75–7.

12. Centers for Disease Control and Prevention. 2010. Frequently asked questions about surgical site infections. http://www.cdc.gov/HAI/ssi/faq_ssi.html (accessed January 27, 2011).

13. Bode L. G. M., J. A. J. W. Kluytmans, H. F. L. Wertheim, D. Bogaers, C. M. J. E. Vandenbroucke-Grauls, R. Roosendaal, A. Troelstra, A. T. Box, A. Voss, I. van der Tweel, et al. 2010. Preventing surgical site infections in nasal carriers of *Staphylococcus aureus*. *N Engl J Med* 362:9–17.

14. Campbell, D. A. Jr., W. G. Henderson, M. J. Englesbe, B. L. Hall, M. O'Reilly, and D. Bratzler. 2008. Surgical site infection prevention: The importance of operative duration and blood transfusion—Results of the first American college of surgeons-national surgical quality improvement program best practices initiative. *J Am Coll Surg* 207:810–20.

15. Kjønniksen, I., B. M. Andersen, V. G. Søndena, L. Segadal. 2002. Preoperative hair removal: A systematic literature review. *AORN J* 75:928–38.

16. Stahel, P. F., A. L. Sabel, M. S. Victoroff, J. Varnell, A. Lembitz, D. J. Boyle, T. J. Clarke, W. R. Smith, and P. S. Mehler. 2010. Wrong-site and wrong-patient procedures in the universal protocol era: Analysis of a prospective database of physician self-reported occurrences. *Arch Surg* 145:978–84.

17. Weber, W. P., W. R. Marti, M. Zwahlen, H. Misteli, R. Rosenthal, S. Reck, and P. Fueglistaler. 2008. The timing of surgical antimicrobial prophylaxis. *Ann Surg* 247:918-26.

18. Dellinger, E. P., S. M. Hausmann, D. W. Bratzler, R. M. Johnson, D. M. Daniel, K. M. Bunt, G. A. Baumgardner, and J. R. Sugarman. 2005. Hospitals collaborate to decrease surgical site infections. *Am J Surg* 190:9-15.

19. de Vries, E. N., L. Dijkstra, S. M. Smorenburg, R. P. Meijer, and M. A. Boermeester. 2010. The surgical patient safety system (SURPASS) checklist optimizes timing of antibiotic prophylaxis. *Patient Saf Surg* 4:6.

20. Ata, A., J. Lee, S. L. Bestle, J. Desemone, and S. C. Stain. 2010. Preoperative hyperglycemia and surgical site infection in general surgery patients. *Arch Surg* 145:858-64.

21. Berg, S. R., F. R. Poritz, K. J. McKenna, D. B. Stewart, and W. A. Koltun. 2011. Risk factors for surgical site infections after colorectal resection in diabetic patients. *J Am Coll Surg* 212:29-34.

22. Dickinson, A., M. Qadan, and H. C. Polk, Jr. 2010. Optimizing surgical care: A contemporary assessment of temperature, oxygen, and glucose. *Am Surg* 76:b571-b577.

23. Anderson, D. J., K. S. Kaye, D. Classen, K. M. Arias, K. Podgorny, H. Burstin, D. P. Calfee, et al. 2008. Strategies to prevent surgical site infections in acute care hospitals. *Infect Control Hosp Epidemiol* 29:S51-S61.

24. Stulberg, J. J., C. P. Delaney, D. V. Neuhauser, D. C. Aron, P. Fu, and S. M. Koroukian. 2010. Adherence to surgical care improvement project measures and the association with postoperative infections. *J Am Med Assoc* 303:2479-85.

25. Lehtinen, S. J., G. Onicescu, K. M. Kuhn, D. J. Cole, and N. F. Esnaola. 2010. Normothermia to prevent surgical site infections after gastrointestinal surgery: Holy grail or false idol? *Ann Surg* 252:696-704.

26. Nurok, M., C. A. Czeisler, L. S. Lehmann. 2010. Sleep deprivation, elective surgical procedures, and informed consent. *N Engl J Med* 363:2577-9.

27. Horan T. C., M. Andrus, and M. A. Dudeck. 2008. CDC/NHSN surveillance definition of healthcare-associated infection and criteria for specific types of infections in the acute care setting. *Am J Infect Control* 36:309-32.

28. Hollenbeak, C. S., J. R. Lave, T. Zeddies, Y. Pei, C. E. Roland, E. F. Sun. 2006. Factors associated with risk of surgical wound infections. *Am J Med Qual* 21-S:29S-34S.

29. Perencevich, E. N., K. E. Sands, S. E. Cosgrove, E. Guadagnoli, E. Meara, and R. Platt. 2003. Health and economic impact of surgical site infections diagnosed after hospital discharge. *Emerg Infect Dis* 9:196-203.

30. Clancy, C. M. 2010. Same-day surgery: What you should know. Agency for Healthcare Research and Quality. http://www.ahrq.gov/consumer/cc/cc040610.htm (accessed January 11, 2011).

CHAPTER 9

1. Barrett, K. E., S. M. Barman, S. Boitano, and H. Brooks. 2010. *Ganong's Review of Medical Physiology.* 23rd ed. New York: McGraw-Hill Companies, Inc.
2. Boyd, S., I. Aggarwal, P. Davey, M. Logan, and D. Nathwani. 2011. Peripheral intravenous catheters: The road to quality improvement and safer patient care. *J Hosp Infect* 77:37–41.
3. Hasselberg, D., B. Ivarsson, R. Andersson, and B. Tingstedt. 2010. The handling of peripheral venous catheters—from non-compliance to evidence-based needs. *J Clin Nurs* 19:3358–63.
4. File, T. M. Jr., and V. L. Abell. 2009. Prevention of bloodstream infections: Basics and beyond. *Crit Care Med* 37:375–6.
5. McHugh, S. M., M. A. Corrigan, B. D. Dimitrov, M. Morris-Downes, F. Fitzpatrick, S. Cowman, S. Tierney, A. D. Hill, and H. Humphreys. 2011. Role of patient awareness in prevention of peripheral vascular catheter-related bloodstream infection. *Infect Control Hosp Epidemiol* 32:95–6.
6. Frequently asked questions about catheters. 2010. Centers for Disease Control and Prevention, http://www.cdc.gov/HAI/bsi/catheter_faqs.html (accessed January 27, 2011).
7. Fahy, B., and M. Sockrider. 2007. American Thoracic Society Patient Information Series: Central venous catheter. *Am J Respir Crit Care Med* 176:P3–P4.
8. English Wikipedia project. Central venous catheter. http://en.wikipedia.org/wiki/Triple-lumen (accessed February 26, 2011).
9. Vallés, J., and R. Ferrer. 2009. Bloodstream infection in the ICU. *Infect Dis Clin North Am* 23:557–69.
10. Pronovost, P. J., C. A. Goeschel, E. Colantuoni, S. Watson, L. H. Lubomski, S. M. Berenholtz, D. A. Thompson, et al. 2010. Sustaining reductions in catheter related bloodstream infections in Michigan intensive care units: Observational study. *Br Med J* 340:c309 (doi: 10.1136/bmj.c309).
11. McGuckin, M., J. Storr, Y. Longtin, B. Allegranzi, and D. Pittet. 2011. Patient empowerment and multimodal hand hygiene promotion: A win-win strategy. *Am J Med Qual* 26:10–7.
12. O'Grady, N. P., M. Alexander, L. A. Burns, E. P. Dellinger, J. Garland, S. O. Heard, P. A. Lipsett, H. Masur, L. A. Mermel, M. L. Pearson, et al.;

Healthcare Infection Control Practices Advisory Committee. 2002. Guidelines for the prevention of intravascular catheter-related infections. Centers for disease control and prevention. *Morb Mortal Wkly Rep Recomm Rep* 51(RR-10):1–29.

13. Centers for Disease Control and Prevention. 2005. Reduction in central line-associated bloodstream infections among patients in intensive care units: Pennsylvania, April 2001-March 2005. *Morb Mortal Wkly Rep (MMWR)* 54:1013–6.

14. Stone, P. W., S. A. Glied, P. D. McNair, N. Matthes, B. Cohen, T. F. Landers, and E. L. Larson. 2010. CMS changes in reimbursements for HAIs: Setting a research agenda. *Med Care* 48:433–9.

15. U.S. Department of Health & Human Services. Hospital Compare, 2010. http://www.hospitalcompare.hhs.gov (accessed February 28, 2011).

16. Centers for Disease Control and Prevention. 2009. First State-Specific Healthcare-Associated Infections Summary Data Report. http://www.cdc.gov/hai/statesummary.html (accessed February 28, 2011).

17. Lipitz-Snyderman, A., D. Steinwachs, D. M. Needham, E. Colantuoni, L. L. Morlock, and P. J. Pronovost. 2011. Impact of a statewide intensive care unit quality improvement initiative on hospital mortality and length of stay: Retrospective comparative analysis. *Br Med J* 342:d219 (doi: 10.1136/bmj.d219).

18. O'Grady, N. P., M. Alexander, L. A. Burns, E. P. Dellinger, J. Garland, S. O. Heard, P. A. Lipsett, H. Masur, L. A. Mermel, M. L. Pearson, et al.; Healthcare Infection Control Practices Advisory Committee. 2011. Guidelines for the prevention of intravascular catheter-related infections. *Clin Infect Dis* 52:3–4 (doi: 10.1093/cid/cir196).

19. Association for Professionals in Injection Control and Epidemiology (APIC). 2009. Guide to the Elimination of Catheter-Related Bloodstream Infections. http://www.apic.org/Content/NavigationMenu/PracticeGuidance/APICEliminationGuides/CRBSI_Elimination_Guide_logo.pdf (accessed February 24, 2011).

20. Rebmann, T., and C. L. Murphy. 2010. Preventing catheter-related bloodstream infections: An executive summary of the APIC elimination guide. *Am J Infect Control* 38:846–48.

CHAPTER 10

1. Russell, T. R. 2008. *I Need an Operation...Now What?* Chicago, IL: American College of Surgeons and Thomson Healthcare.

2. Williams, W. W., J. Mariano, M. Spurrier, H. D. Donnell Jr., R. L. Breckenridge Jr., R. L. Anderson, I. K. Wachsmuth, C. Thornsberry,

D. R. Graham, D. W. Thibeault, et al. 1984. Nosocomial meningitis due to citrobacter diversus in neonates: New aspects of the epidemiology. *J Infect Dis* 150:229–35.

3. Lopez, J., J. DiLiberto, and M. McGuckin. 1988. *Am J Infect Control* 16:26–9.
4. Christ, P. The ten infection control commandments of child day care. http://www.centraliowachildcare.org/healthconsulting/tencommandmentschildcare.pdf (accessed November 3 2011).
5. Meadows, E., and N. Le Saux. 2004. A systematic review of the effectiveness of antimicrobial rinse-free hand sanitizers for prevention of illness-related absenteeism in elementary school children. *BMC Public Health* 4:50 (doi:10.1186/1471-2458-4.50).
6. Bloom, B., and R. A. Cohen. 2009. Summary health statistics for U.S. children: National health interview survey, 2007. National center for health statistics. *Vital Health Stat* 10(239):1–80. http://www.cdc.gov/nchs/data/series/sr_10/sr10_239.pdf (accessed April 22 2011).
7. The Children's Health Initiative. 2009. San Diego county report card on children and families. http://www.thechildrensinitiative.org/reportcard.htm (accessed April 22 2011).
8. Guinan, M., M. McGuckin, and A. Sevareid. 1997. Who washes hands after using the bathroom? *Am J Infect Control* 25:424–5.
9. Guinan, M., and M. McGuckin. 2002. The effect of a comprehensive handwashing program on absenteeism in elementary schools. *Am J Infect Control* 30:217–20.
10. Health and safety statistics 2009/10. The health and safety executive, annual astatistics report. United Kingdom: HSE Books. http://www.hse.gov.uk/statistics (accessed March 11 2011).
11. Hübner NO, C. Hübner, M. Wodny, G. Kampf, A. Kramer. 2010. Effectiveness of alcohol-based hand disinfectants in a public administration: Impact on health and work performance related to acute respiratory symptoms and diarrhea. *BMC Infect Dis* 10:250 (doi:10.1186/1471-2334-10-250).
12. Gerba, C. P. 2001. Workplace germ study fact sheet. The Clorox co. http://www.onsitecomputercleaning.ca/cloroxstudy.pdf (accessed March 11 2011).
13. Centers for Medicare and Medicaid Services. 2009. American recovery and reinvestment act: Ambulatory surgical center healthcare-associated infection (ASC-HAI) Prevention Initiative. https://www.cms.gov/certificationandcomplianc/02_ascs.asp (accessed April 27 2011).
14. Schaefer, M. K., M. Jhung, M. Dahl, S. Schillie, C. Simpson, E. Llata, R. Link-Gelles, R. Sinkowitz-Cochran, P. Patel, E. Bolyard, et al. 2010.

Infection control assessment of ambulatory surgical centers. *J Am Med Assoc* 303:2273-9.

15. Barie, P. S. 2010. Editorial: Infection control assessment of ambulatory surgical centers. *J Am Med Assoc* 303:2295-7.

16. Ambulatory Surgery Center Association. Ambulatory surgery centers: A positive trend in healthcare. http://www.ascassociation.org/advocacy/AmbulatorySurgeryCentersPositiveTrendHealthCare.pdf (accessed March 11 2011).

17. Clancy, C. M. 2010. Same-day surgery: What you should know. Agency for Healthcare Research and Quality, April 6. http://www.ahrq.gov/consumer/cc/cc040610.htm (accessed May 3 2010).

18. Harrison, P. L., P. A Hara, J. E. Pope, M. C. Young, E. Y. Rula. 2011. The impact of postdischarge telephonic follow-up on hospital readmissions. *Popul Health Manag* 14:27-32.

19. Jencks, S. F., M. V. Williams, and E. A. Coleman. 2009. Rehospitalizations among patients in the medicare fee-for-service program. *N Engl J Med* 360:1418-28.

20. Kane, R. 2011. Finding the right level of posthospital care: "We didn't realize there was any other option for him." *J Am Med Assoc* 305:284-93.

21. Patel, A. S, M. B. White-Comstock, C. D. Woolard, and J. F Perz. 2009. Infection control practices in assisted living facilities: A response to hepatitis B virus infection outbreaks. *Infect Control Hosp Epidemiol* 30:209-14.

22. The Assisted Living Federation of America. 2009. "Guide to choosing an assisted living community." http://www.alfa.org/alfa/Checklist_for_Evaluating_Communities.asp.

23. Centers for Disease Control and Prevention. 2011. Notes from the field: Deaths from acute hepatitis B virus infection associated with assisted blood glucose monitoring in an assisted-living facility—North Carolina, August-October 2010. *MMWR Morb Mortal Wkly Rep* 60:182.

24. Phillips, L. R., and G. Guo. 2011. Mistreatment in assisted living facilities: Complaints, substantiations, and risk factors. *Gerontologist* 51:343-53.

25. American Healthcare Association Research Department. Long Term Care (LTC) Statistics: Nursing facility patient characteristics report. Updated March 2011. http://www.ahcancal.org/research_data/oscar_data/Pages/default.aspx (accessed March 18 2011).

26. Smith, P. W., G. Bennett, S. Bradley, P. Drinka, E. Lautenbach, J. Marx, L. Mody, L. Nicolle, K. Stevenson. 2008. SHEA/APIC Guideline: Infection prevention and control in the long-term care facility. *Infect Control Hosp Epidemiol* 29:785-814.

27. Strausbaugh, L. J., and C. L. Joseph. 2000. The burden of infection in long-term care. *Infect Control Hospital Epidemiol* 21:674–9.
28. Strausbaugh, L. J., S. R. Sukumar, and C. L. Joseph. 2003. Infectious disease outbreaks in nursing homes: An unappreciated hazard for frail elderly persons. *Clin Infect Dis* 36:870–6.
29. Utsumi, M., K. Makimoto, N. Quroshi, and N. Ashida. 2010. Types of infectious outbreaks and their impact in elderly care facilities: A review of the literature. *Age and Ageing* 39:299–305.
30. McGuckin, M., and J. Brown. 2004. Validations of a comprehensive infection control program. *Director* 12:14–7.

CHAPTER 11

1. Guinan, J. L., M. McGuckin, A. Shubin, and J. Tighe. 2005. A descriptive review of malpractice claims for healthcare-associated infections in Philadelphia. *Am J Infect Control* 33:310–2.
2. Mello, M. M., C. Amitabh, A. A. Gawande, and D. M. Studdert. 2010. National costs of the medical liability system. *Health Aff (Millwood)* 29:1569–77.
3. Sharpe, V. A. 2003. Special supplement: Promoting patient safety: An ethical basis for policy deliberation. *Hastings Cent Rep* 33:S1–S20.
4. Hallinan, J. T. 2004. Suite wrinkle: In malpractice trials, juries rarely have the last word. Wall Street Journal, November 30, 2004 at A1.
5. Jasper, M. C. 2001. *The Law of Medical Malpractice*. 2nd ed. 27. Dobbs Ferry, NY: Oceana Publications.
6. Eades, R. W. 1998. *Jury Instructions on Damages in Tort Actions*. 4th ed., 298. Lexis Law Publishing.
7. Relis, T. 2006. "It's not about the money!" A theory on misconceptions of plaintiff's litigation aims. *Univ Pittsbg Law Rev* 68:341–85.
8. Gallagher T. H., Waterman A. D., Ebers, A. G., Fraser, V. J., and Levinson, W. 2003. Patients' and physicians' attitudes regarding the disclosure of medical errors. *J Am Med Assoc* 289:1001–7.
9. Mazor, K. M., S. R. Simon, R. A. Yood, Martinson, B. C., Gunter, M. J., Reed G. W., and Gurwitz, J. H. 2004. Health plan members' views about disclosure of medical errors. *Ann Intern Med* 140:409–18.
10. COPIC insurance Company. 3Rs Program. http://www.callcopic.com/home/what-we-offer/coverages/medical-professional-liability-insurance-co/physicians-medical-practices/special-programs/3rs-program/ (accessed March 11, 2011).
11. CAL. EVID. CODE 1160 (Supp 2004).

12. FLA. STAT.ANN. CH. 90.4026 (Supp 2004).
13. MASS. GEN. LAWS CH. 233, §23D.
14. TEX. CIV. PRAC. & REM. CODE ANN. §18.061 (Supp 2004-05).
15. Dauer, E. A., and L. J. Marcus. 1997. Adapting mediation to link resolution of medical malpractice disputes with healthcare quality improvement. *Law Contemp Probl* 60:185–218.
16. Blatt R., M. Brown, and J. Lerner. Co-mediation: A success story at Chicago's Rush Medical Center. http://www.adrsystems.com/news/Co-Mediation.pdf (accessed March 15, 2011).
17. Lee A., L. A, Rosengard, and M. Parker. 2004. "Committing to Mediation: Enriched Resolution of Medical Malpractice Actions for Patients, Doctors, and Insurance Companies." The Intelligencer.
18. Jenkins R. C., L. A. Warren, and N. Gravenstein. 2010. Mandatory pre-suit mediation: Local malpractice reform benefiting patients and healthcare providers. *J Healthc Risk Manag* 30:27–35.
19. American Arbitration Association. Non-binding arbitration rules for consumer disputes and business disputes. January 1, 2010. http://www.adr.org/sp.asp?id=35917 (accessed March 15, 2011).
20. Mello, M. M., and T. H. Gallagher. 2010. Malpractice reform—Opportunities for leadership by healthcare institutions and liability insurers. *N Engl J Med* 362:1353-6.
21. Kraman, S. S., and G. Hamm. 1999. Risk management: Extreme honesty may be the best policy. *Ann Intern Med* 131:963-7.
22. The Joint Commission. Hospital accreditation. http://www.jointcommission.org/accreditation/hospitals.aspx (accessed March 11, 2011).
23. The Joint Commission. Report a complaint. http://www.jointcommission.org/GeneralPublic/Complaint/ (accessed March 11, 2011).
24. Annas, G. J. 2006. The patient's right to safety--Improving the quality of care through litigation against hospitals. *N Engl J Med* 354:2063-6.
25. Thompson v. Nason Hospital, 527 Pa. 330, 591 (1991).
26. Berwick, D. M., D. R, Calkins, C. J, McCannon, and A. D. Hachbarth. 2006. The 100,000 Lives Campaign: Setting a goal and a deadline for improving healthcare quality. *J Am Med Assoc* 295:324-7.
27. Mello, M. M., and T. A. Brennan. 2002. Deterrence of medical errors: Theory and evidence for malpractice reform. *Texas L Rev* 80:1595-637.
28. Sage, W. M., J. G, Zivlin, and N. B. Chase. 2006. Bridging the relational-regulatory gap: A pragmatic information policy for the patient safety and medical practice. *Vanderbilt Law Rev* 59:1284-5.
29. Pub. Citizen, Inc. v. Dep't of Health and Human Servs., 332 F.3d 854, 663 (2003).

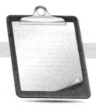

Resources

Accreditation Association for Ambulatory Healthcare website explains standards that ambulatory facilities must meet to obtain accreditation (www.aaahc.org).

Agency for Healthcare Research and Quality (AHRQ). *Federal Agency Working to Improve Quality, Safety, Efficiency, and Effectiveness of Healthcare.* www.ahrq.gov; also see *Same-Day Surgery: What you should know,* http://www.ahrq.gov/consumer/cc/cc040610.htm, and *Taking Care of Myself: A guide for when I leave the hospital* (http://www.ahrq.gov/qual/goinghomeguide.pdf).

Ambulatory Surgery Center Association website provides details about quality and safety regulations (www.ascassociation.org).

American Hospital Association provides online information about hospital patients' rights and responsibilities and steps patients can take to ensure safer care and good communication with their healthcare workers (www.aha.org).

American Medical Association website helps users to find a doctor and check doctors' credentials (www.ama-assn.org).

Assisted Living Federation of America's *Guide to Choosing an Assisted Living Community* (http://www.alfa.org/images/alfa/PDFs/PublicationsResources/Guide_to_Choosing_Assisted_Living_Community.pdf).

Campaign Zero™ offers simple explanations about common hospital hazards and easy checklists to help families safeguard their loved ones' care in the hospital (http://www.campaignzero.org).

Centers for Disease Control and Prevention, Division of Healthcare Quality Promotion, Blog: Preventing Infections in Healthcare Settings (http://blogs.cdc.gov/safehealthcare/); also see the website on healthcare-associated infections (HAIs) with links to consumer information and FAQs about each type of infection (http://www.cdc.gov/hai/), and *Infection Control in Long-Term Care Facilities* (http://www.cdc.gov/HAI/settings/ltc_settings.html).

Center for Medicare and Medicaid Services (CMS). A division of the Department of Health and Human Services which finances and administers the Medicare and Medicaid programs and establishes standards for the operation of healthcare facilities that receive funds under the Medicare or Medicaid programs. This website will help you to find hospitals and other facilities in your area, compare them, and to add your own observations, www.hospitalcompare.hhs.gov/; to compare nursing homes (http://www.medicare.gov/NHCompare/Include/DataSection/Questions/SearchCriteriaNEW.asp).

COPIC Insurance Company: 3Rs Program, to promote communication and assistance from physicians for patients who experience a medical injury (www.callcopic.com).

Department of Health and Human Services' *Healthfinder* helps people find doctors and health facilities (www.healthfinder.gov).

Empowered Patient Coalition. Non-profit private organization promoting patient advocates and patient rights, and helping educate people on patient safety issues (www.empoweredpatientcoalition.org).

Federation of State Medical Boards' website lets consumers check doctors' education and credentials and lists any disciplinary action against each doctor (www.FSMB.org).

Health Grades publishes reports and ratings to help consumers to choose the best doctors and hospitals (www.healthgrades.com).

Joint Commission. If you have a complaint about the quality of care at an accredited hospital, go to http://www.jointcommission.org and fill out their simple complaint form; to download a form on accredited nursing homes in your search area, go to http://www.jointcommission.org/facts_about_long_term_care_accreditation; also go to the Commission's Quality Check® website www.qualitycheck.org for ratings and information about all types of medical facilities and "grades" showing how the facility compares to similar institutions.

Josie King Foundation provides information on patient safety, tips on staying safe, and a message board where people can post stories and ask/answer questions about patient safety issues (www.josieking.org).

McGuckin Methods International provides ongoing educational resources for consumers as well as healthcare are providers (www.hhreports.com)

Medicana's website includes videos of medical examinations and procedures related to all aspects of healthcare, including surgeries, birth, catheter insertion, and more (www.medicanalife.com).

National Foundation for Infectious Diseases publishes print and online fact sheets and educational materials for consumers about the causes, treatment and prevention of infectious diseases (www.nfid.org).

National Patient Safety Foundation conducts research programs and safety awareness conferences. Their website lists links to medical information sources for consumers (www.npsf.org).

Next Step in Care provides easy-to-use guides to help family caregivers manage post-hospital care (www.nextstepincare.org).

Patient Safety Group works with hospitals throughout the U.S. to improve patient safety and healthcare quality (www.patientsafetygroup.org).

Rate MDs helps consumers find a doctor or dentist who has been rated by other consumers. Users can also enter their own ratings (www.ratemds.com).

Safe Care Campaign website provides videos, downloadable brochures, and infection prevention facts and tips for consumers (www.safecarecampaign.org).

Safe Patient Project, a Consumers Union campaign focused on eliminating medical harm, improving FDA oversight of prescription drugs, and promoting disclosure laws that give information to consumers about healthcare safety and quality, includes a blog, stories shared by patients harmed by healthcare and healthcare-associated infection statistics reports on hospitals in 25 states (www.safepatientproject.org).

The American College of Surgeons' website explains surgical operations, tests, medications, and pain management (http://www.facs.org/patienteducation/index.html).

Yoursurgery.com website presents easy to understand explanations, diagrams, and animated videos of common surgical procedures (www.yoursurgery.com).

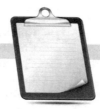

Index

Wallet Card: Take This to the Hospital with You

One for You, One for a Friend or Loved One

✄- -

Healthcare-Associated Infection Insurance Card

Remember, When Hospitalized ...

- Make sure you have a daily bath.
- Tell all healthcare workers and visitors to wash or sanitize their hands.
- Tell your doctor if you have recently been: hospitalized, admitted to a nursing home, exposed to or treated for MRSA, or currently have an infection (for example, urinary tract).
- Identify an advocate and understand the use of "rapid response."

(cont.)

✄- -

Healthcare-Associated Infection Insurance Card

Remember, When Hospitalized ...

- Make sure you have a daily bath.
- Tell all healthcare workers and visitors to wash or sanitize their hands.
- Tell your doctor if you have recently been: hospitalized, admitted to a nursing home, exposed to or treated for MRSA, or currently have an infection (for example, urinary tract).
- Identify an advocate and understand the use of "rapid response."

(cont.)

- Discuss informed consent and ask your surgeon about infection rates and antibiotics.
- Check your skin around an IV for any redness or swelling.
- Urinary catheters should only be used when necessary, not for convenience.
- After discharge, check your wound site for any redness, swelling, or drainage if you have pain.

©MMI, Inc. 2004, Ardmore, PA; www.hhreports.com

- Discuss informed consent and ask your surgeon about infection rates and antibiotics.
- Check your skin around an IV for any redness or swelling.
- Urinary catheters should only be used when necessary, not for convenience.
- After discharge, check your wound site for any redness, swelling, or drainage if you have pain.

©MMI, Inc. 2004, Ardmore, PA; www.hhreports.com

HAND HYGIENE TECHNIQUE WITH SOAP AND WATER

🕐 **Duration of the entire procedure: 40-60 seconds**

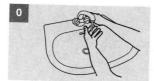

0 Wet hands with water

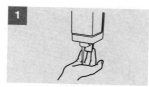

1 Apply enough soap to cover all hand surface

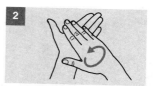

2 Rub hands palm to palm

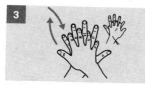

3 Right palm over left dorsum with interlaced fingers and vice versa

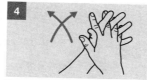

4 Palm to palm with fingers interlaced

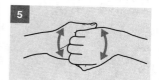

5 Backs of fingers to opposing palms with fingers interlocked

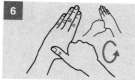

6 Rotational rubbing of left thumb clasped in right palm and vice versa

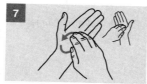

7 Rotational rubbing, backward and forward with clasped fingers of right hand in left palm and vice versa

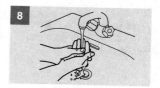

8 Rinse hands with water

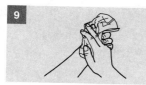

9 Dry hands throughly with a single use towel

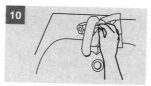

10 Use towel to turn off faucet

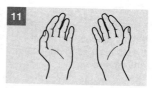

11 Your hands are now safe.

(WHO Guidelines on Hand Hygiene in Healthcare. WHO, 2009.)

HAND HYGIENE TECHNIQUE WITH HAND SANITIZER

🕐 **Duration of the entire procedure: 20-30 seconds**

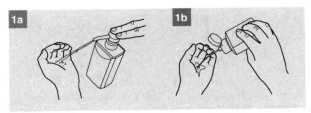

Apply a palmful of the product in a cupped hand, covering all surfaces

Rub hands palm to palm

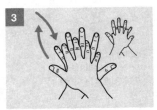

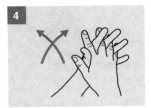

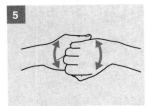

Right palm over left dorsum with interlaced fingers and vice versa

Palm to palm with fingers interlaced

Backs of fingers to opppos-ing palms with fingers interlocked

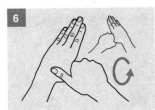

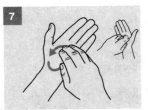

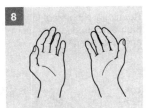

Rotational rubbing of left thumb clasped in right palm and vice versa

Rotational rubbing, backward and forward with clasped fingers of right hand in left palm and vice versa

Once dry, your hands are safe.

(WHO Guidelines on Hand Hygiene in Healthcare, 2009.)